Publisher's address:

10336 Loch Lomond Rd.

Middletown, CA 95461

CONTENTS

FOREWORD

Several healthy young friends were so devastated by Dengue infections that it scared me into changing my lifestyle and writing this book. I can't afford such a severe health setback, particularly when it's preventable.

Dengue infections are rarely fatal – re-infections are more so – but each case takes an average 17 days out of our lives and those of friends, relatives and caregivers. Multiply that by the 400 million of us who will contract Dengue this year and we'll collectively lose 18 *million* productive, happy years. Unnecessarily.

Dealing With Dengue reduces your chances of infection by 99% and tells you and your doctor what to do if an *Aedes Eegypti* mosquito gets her proboscis into you.

1. WHAT NOT TO DO...

By Jodi Ettenberg

I have tried to avoid writing about myself other than in the abstract. I love sharing what I eat and learn, and the stories of food and people involve me in some way as it is a personal blog. But I don't want my blog to be a place where I whine or rant. I want it to be a place where people can learn through food.

So when I started losing clumps of hair in February last year I neither wrote about it nor shared updates on my Facebook page. A month later, when I stopped being able to bend my hands or knees without pain or look at bright light, I didn't mention that either. I kept up my usual schedule in Vietnam, exploring the Mekong and surrounding regions and walking around town for hours a day.

In May, after flying to England to visit my brother, I could barely walk down the street without feeling exhausted. Alarmingly, when my leg or arm was itchy and I scratched it I'd develop lines of bruises, coloring the spot where nails met skin. As the summer went on and my existing obligations and plans were ticked off the list -- conferences, meetups, interviews and more -- I found myself getting more tired and sick. My immune system was not cooperating with anything I did; every cold or virus seemed to latch onto me stubbornly and most of my days were obfuscated by a cloud of exhaustion.

Doctors were fairly unhelpful. One suggested that I was just stressed. As a former corporate lawyer I was pretty intimate with high stress situations, and I certainly was not stressed – except about the fact that my health was deteriorating. Which was, I think, pretty reasonable on the spectrum of

Events to Stress About. In actuality, the pain and hair loss had started at a time when I was the least stressed in decades; I was in Vietnam, loving my exploration of the city and its soups. Another doctor thought I had lupus and, to be fair, many of the symptoms lined up, but blood tests gave no indication of lupus. So back to square one.

I confided in my close friends who stretched their arms wide to pull in connections from their broader networks in hope of helping me figure out what was wrong. I was introduced to, and corresponded with, a woman whose many symptoms led her to cut a number of significant foods from her diet and completely change the way she lives her life in an attempt to keep her pain under control. I met a gentleman at a conference who had similar health issues while trying to grow a startup, leading him to temporarily walk away from his company while he focused on getting better, a terribly tough decision to make. And I was given a book recommendation that calmed my brain down considerably, Full Catastrophe Living, written for those dealing with the stress and exhaustion of chronic pain and fortuitously updated days before it was suggested to me.

By October, when I was heading to India with my mother, I felt like I was hanging on by a thread. I sat in a pile of clothes packing, in tears. I was happy to be taking her to a country she wanted to see but feeling like I might just stop functioning somewhere between Jaipur and Agra and fall into a deep, long sleep.

We did have a terrific time in India, exploring the chaos and color of Rajasthan in a few too-short weeks. But I did still get sick again and again, and much of the trip is cloudy with pain, too. By the time I flew home to Canada, the airline stewardesses took one look at me as we boarded the plane and then cleared out the back row and insisted I sleep. I was tired and confused and tired of being tired and confused.

Then I figured it out.

I kept going back to February when it all began. Earlier in the month I was supposed to go to the Mekong, but I woke up feeling so sick and tired that I couldn't budge. I had a splitting headache and it felt like someone was pressing on my eyeballs; nothing relieved the pain. I thought I had a bad flu and I postponed my visit. My "flu" cleared up a few days later for the most part, though the headache took longer to go away. A few days later, when I was visiting Vung Tau with my friends, I developed a strange rash all over my stomach. It wasn't itchy -- it was just flat red dots that appeared in constellations all over my torso and around my belly button. I remember my friends all staring at my stomach one morning, confused as to what was causing it. We went with heat rash, and quickly forgot it. A few days later it was gone.

What could have caused the rash and my flu-like symptoms and then all the tiredness, joint issues and pain?

Dengue.

Interestingly, that's exactly whymy friends were in Vietnam -- they had gotten Dengue in Bangkok and were in recovery on their visa run. I Googled "Dengue rash stomach" and saw exactly what was on my stomach in Vung Tau. Then I looked into what happens when you don't take care of yourself when you have Dengue. (Those who have experience with it will know that the disease is not really treated per se; treatment involves hospital visits, hydration, rest and monitoring white blood cells and platelets, both of which are dangerously low when in the grasp of the Dengue virus).

I learned that, when you ignore it as I did, it wreaks havoc on your immune system, your joints, and on your general state of being. I went to a tropical diseases doctor and presented my case, and he confirmed that a Dengue infection is almost certainly what I'd contracted, especially given a February infection and my subsequent blood test results, which showed a lower-than-normal white blood cell and platelet count.

There's little to do at this point other than listen to what my body tells me, resting more, staying out late less, keeping the long haul flights to a minimum. (The time zone changes and effects on your body's adrenal system were, my doctor said, particularly problematic for long hauls.) And, you know, avoiding mosquitoes to the extent possible. Damn you, mosquitos!

So, after many months of saying nothing I'm writing to reiterate what not to do when you get Dengue. Or, put another way, when in Dengue-prone areas and having symptoms of the flu, if you see a rash on your person GET THEE TO A DOCTOR. I wish I had gone to check it out and could have then taken care of myself properly.– Jodi blogs charmingly at Legal Nomads.

2. WHAT IS DENGUE?

On an average, between 14.8 and 18.9 days are lost as the patient is incapacitated or a family member needs to stay at home to care for
Dengue-infected children or relatives. – Red Cross Report, 2014

Dengue is a Spanish word meaning 'well-dressed, or 'a dandy'. We use it to label the disease but no one is quite sure why. The most popular explanation is that when Spanish slaves in the West Indies contracted Dengue they were described as having the posture and gait of a dandy, and the disease was known for a while as "dandy fever".

Dengue, or *Dengue fever*, is caused by a virus carried by the female *Aedes aegypti* mosquito. She feeds on your blood in the early morning and late afternoon and breeds indoors in cool, dark corners.

Half of all Dengue-infected people have mild symptoms but, for the other half, it's a painful, debilitating, and potentially fatal disease.

A minority of people – usually previously infected – develop a complicated, hemorrhagic form of Dengue, known as *Dengue Hemorrhagic Fever*, or *Dengue Shock Syndrome*. Scientists now call it *Severe Dengue*. Severe Dengue is a leading cause of serious illness and death among children in some Asian and Latin American countries. World wide, 12,000 people die of it every year. Thailand, where I live, has extensive experience with Dengue and a good public health system so our mortality rate is less than 1%. But it requires immediate hospitalization, fluid replacement and sometimes blood transfusions.

The global incidence of Dengue has grown dramatically as our planet has warmed. Half of the world's population is now at risk, especially those of us living in urban and suburban areas in the tropics and subtropics. There is no vaccine yet to prevent Dengue, and no 'cure' for its symptoms. You have to manage dengue's symptoms and let it run its course. Recognizing the symptoms promptly and treating them correctly makes a life-saving difference.

3. DIAGNOSING DENGUE

People experience a combination of symptoms associated with Dengue. Here, in decreasing order of frequency, are the most common:

1. Sudden, high fever up to 41°C (105.8°F) for 2–7 days.

2. Severe pain behind your eyes and when you move your eyes

3. Intense headache

4. Impaired judgement (like drunkenness; can't concentrate)

5. Persistent vomiting, diarrhea.

6. Abdominal pain or tenderness

7. Feeling sick and being sick

8. Severe pain in your bones and joints (it was called *breakbone* fever!)

9. Severe muscle pain in your lower back, arms and legs during the first hours of illness.

10. Extreme tiredness

11. Loss of appetite

12. Chills, shivering

13. Sore throat

14. Metallic taste in your mouth

15. Red eyes.

16. Small, flat, red spots forming a rash

17. Minor bleeding from nose and gums

18. Blood in your urine

19. Red rash on your palms and soles.

20. Easy bruising

21. Flushing: a pale pink face rash that then disappears.

22. Swollen lymph nodes in the neck and groin.

23. Fluid accumulation

24. Enlarged liver

25. Relatively low heart rate (bradycardia) and

26. Low blood pressure (hypotension).

27. Low white cell count

You may experience either a few or many of these in any combination. Any three suggests Dengue infection. Sudden, high fever is the most important clue.

Dengue affects everyone differently. Most infected people, especially kids and teens, experience mild or no symptoms. People with symptoms typically suffer them for 2–3 weeks but some endure them for months or years. A Swiss friend who was infected in India in 2009 was still feeling the symptoms in 2014. Some, especially infants, die.

- Diagnosing Dengue is tricky because your symptoms often resembles the 'flu. Then they develop to resemble diseases like West Nile Virus or chikungunya.

- You should see your GP if you develop fever- or flu-like symptoms within two weeks of returning from an area where the Dengue virus is common – such as Latin America, the Southern States of the USA, South East Asia, the Far East and the Indian subcontinent. Tell him you suspect dengue.There is little your GP can do to alter the course of the infection but it's important to get your condition diagnosed in case your symptoms become more ominous.

- Even if your symptoms are mild you'll experience discomfort *and* you should spend a few days resting at home. This will reduce the risk of your spreading the virus and help you recover quicker.

When Should I Seek Medical Advice?

Most people recover in 2–3 weeks but sometimes symptoms worsen and can become life-threatening *Severe Dengue.* Severe Dengue is a potentially deadly complication.

Severe Dengue warning signs occur 3–7 days after the first symptoms. The next 24–48 hours of the critical stage can be lethal.

Get proper medical care to avoid complications and risk of death. Go **IMMEDIATELY** to an emergency room or the closest health care provider if, in the course of a suspected Dengue infection, you see these warning signs:

- Decreased temperature (below 38°C/ 100°F)
- Pale, cold, or clammy skin
- Blood vessels damaged or leaky
- The number of clot-forming cells (platelets) in your blood drops
- Severe abdominal pain
- Persistent vomiting
- Red spots or rashes on your skin
- Your palms and soles become bright red and swollen.
- Your nose or gums bleed
- Vomiting blood
- Black, tarry stools (feces)
- Drowsiness, fatigue, or irritability
- Difficulty breathing
- Rapid breathing
- Problems with your lungs, liver and heart
- Shock (collapsing due to internal fluid loss)

There's lots more to be said because the symptoms and their permutations are so varied, but it would fill many pages. I've started a video channel on YouTube devoted to case histories, so you can see the variation in people's symptoms. There's a website, www.dengue.us, with a forum and other stuff about Dengue, too.

4. TREATMENT

There is no specific treatment and no antiviral drugs specifically for Dengue. But it's **vitally important that you treat the *symptoms* of Dengue!** Here's what to do:

1. If you're in pain, use painkillers with acetaminophen (Tylenol, *et al.*) only.

2. Read the *Painkillers* chapter in this book and prevent liver damage.

3. Read the *Traditional Chinese Medicine* chapter and repair liver damage.

4. Reduce high fevers (>104°F or 40°C) with cool compresses or lukewarm baths.

5. Rest, rest, rest. And rest. Did I mention *rest*?

6. Drink plenty of fluids to prevent dehydration.

7. To protect those around you, completely prevent mosquito bites while you're feverish.

8. **If you start feeling worse in the first 24 hours after your fever goes down, go to hospital immediately** to be checked for complications.

9. Remember: convalescence is slow and **people often feel depressed** for weeks afterwards.

10. **Drink as much water** as you can in order to replace fluid loss. It will also help to bring down your body temperature.

11. **Avoid solid foods** until the fever is gone. Drink plenty of distilled water, juices and smoothies.

Painkillers & Blood Thinners

If you suspect a Dengue infection, avoid painkillers containing ibuprofen, Naproxen, aspirin, aspirin-containing drugs or NSAIDs (Alleve, Motrin, Advil, etc). Use Tylenol for pain.

Do NOT take blood thinners like Warfarin/Coumadin. Blood thinners can trigger the bleeding typical of Severe Dengue. If you're taking blood thinners like Coumadin (warfarin) or Methotrexate, contact your physician to see if you should stop temporarily.

Read the *Painkillers and Your Liver* chapter later in this book. It's probably the most long-term useful advice in the entire book.

Emergency Suggestions for Physicians

Your local physician may be unfamiliar with Dengue so take this book with you and show her the *Dengue for MDs* chapter. It's up to date with WHO and CDC guidelines and may save valuable time. Or download and print out one of the PDFs on the Dengue Website.

5. FOLK REMEDIES

Here are some natural remedies from around the world. Try them for 1–2 days and always consult your doctor if you notice anything out of the ordinary. There's no solid clinical evidence that any of them are effective but absence of scientific proof has never stopped anyone. Please, please, email me at godfree@dengue.us and let me know your experience with them.

Papaya Leaf Juice. Folks here in Thailand swear by papaya leaf juice. It's so popular that a guy bottles and delivers it all over town during the monsoon. Friends who've used it claim it stopped their platelet count from dropping. Field trials of the efficacy of papaya leaf juice on platelet count look promising, too. Better still, it's free and there seem to be no contra-indications – except that it tastes bad – just as medicines are supposed to! Here's how to whip up glass of awful-tasting papaya leaf juice:

- Pick two young, light-green leaves from the top of your papaya tree.
- Discard the stems and larger veins
- Pound the leaves in a mortar and pestle or toss them into the blender with a cup of water.
- Your two leaves will yield about two tablespoons (30 ml) of juice – sufficient for a day's sipping.
- Drink it fresh and raw. And yes, it really does taste awful.

Tulsi (Basil Leaves): Bitter, pungent basil leaf tea has been used for centuries to lower body temperature and strengthen the immune system. Chew 10-15 basil leaves twice a day or boil them in 200ml water on low heat until half the water boils off, then sip the tea 2-3 times a day.

Kakamachi leaves help reduce fever. In India you can buy Kakamachi syrup as a soothing, cooling drink or prepare a decoction of fresh and dried leaves. 2 cups/day.

Neem leaves, Neem Oil: Neem is an all-round disinfectant. Try 30 ml. of neem leaf tea 3x/day.

Fruits Rich in Vitamin C are general immunotonifiers and help you absorb iron.

Coriander Leaves: Long used to bring down fevers, coriander leaves can be chewed fresh, juiced, or decocted. 10 ml. of fresh coriander leaf juice 2x/day.

Chyavanprash, an Ayurvedic recipe for a sweet jam-like tonic that can be taken as it is an immunobooster, blood purifier and general tonifier. Available at most Indian grocery stores. Kids like it on toast.

Cassia Root: Another traditional tonic and fever-reducer.

Fenugreek leaf tea: Yet another traditional tonic and fever-reducer.

Bloodwort: Prescribed by Ayurvedic physicians for most fevers. As a hot infusion it brings out sweat and reduces the fever. Note that *it also lowers blood pressure*, so check your blood pressure before trying it.

Fresh, unchilled watermelon juice. A Singapore TCM practitioner recommends it.

Pink Guava Juice – Cell wall strengthening, high in iron and vitamin C. Used for treating Dengue in Indonesia.

Pomegranate + black grape juice helps circulatory blood flow.

Orange juice helps with cooling, digestion, increased urinary output, and promotes antibodies for faster healing and recovery.

Red Date and Red Yeast Tea. Another Indonesian Dengue favorite.

Coconut Water. Cooling, replenishes electrolytes and trace minerals.

Isotonic Drinks. These are chemical, usually in cans, and taste bland. But they are safe and effective.

Bitter Gourd and Frog Leg Soup. Malaysian Chinese swear by this bitter soup. It's *really* bitter!

Crab Soup (Sup Ketam). A strong-smelling Malaysian favorite for recuperation.

Palm Dates. High in sugar, zinc, vitamins and calmative to intestinal disturbances. Buy the highest quality you can find and suck on them.

Fu Fang Compound E-Jiao Jiang. A traditional Chinese tonic formula with several contra-indications. Check with your TCM doctor before taking it.

Treating Dengue Rash

If it's itchy, these traditional anti-itch (antipruritic) remedies will give you fast, fast relief:

- **Calamine Lotion.** CVS brand is best.

- **Oatmeal baths.** *Avena sativa.* The oats you eat for breakfast. Very soothing.

- **Peppermint.** *Mentha piperita.* Add a few drops of peppermint oil to corn flour and apply directly to the itchy area.

- **Chickweed.** *Stellaria media.* In creams at health food stores.

- **Witch Hazel** *Hamamelis virginiana.* From most drug stores. Apply direct.

6. CHILDREN & DENGUE

Every 25 minutes a child's life is lost to Dengue – The Red Cross

Although we speak of 'making a full recovery' from disease, we rarely do. All serious diseases are permanent setbacks. We never fully make up the lost time. energy, and invisible damage to our systems. That's why diseases we *can* prevent, like Dengue, should be high on our child care to-do list.

We often fail to notice a first infection in younger children. They, and most folks with a first Dengue infection, generally have a milder illness than older children and adults – so their first infection often goes undiagnosed.

Dengue is more likely to develop into Severe Dengue (formerly called Dengue hemorrhagic fever) if there's been a previous infection. *That's* why babies and young children are at increased risk of this complication: they may have been infected once before without anyone even noticing.

Diagnosing Dengue in Young Children

If there have been reports of Dengue in your area and your child has a fever and skin rashes or aching joints, **contact your doctor immediately**. The symptoms of Dengue and chikungunya (another *aedes*-borne disease) are similar, so your doctor may order a blood test to confirm her diagnosis. It's often hard to guess what ails young children, so here are a few clues to add to the symptom list:

- Is your child playful? An energy drop is an early sign.
- Look for weakness and sleepiness.
- Does he have a headache? In 99% of cases, this is the first sign – days before rashes, etc.,

appear.

- Does he have a fever?

- Dengue fevers in children generally run above 100F (38C).

- If the fever subsides but he's still not playful, then he may have Dengue.

- Lab tests usually won't show Dengue infection for the first 3 days, so his health depends on your powers of observation.

Treating Children's Symptoms

- Treat your kid's symptoms like your own, with a few important differences.

- Isolate him from any possibility of mosquito bites. He's highly infectious and could infect your whole household.

- Reduce or eliminate activities like running around. Have him rest in bed.

- Give him light, nourishing food.

- Give him plenty of fluids. Dengue causes leaky blood vessels and increases water loss:
    - 12 months old or over 22lb. (10 kg) should drink at least 1 qt/l /day.
    - Over 88lb. (40 kg) should drink at least 2 quarts/liter a day.

- Put a wet cloth on his forehead every so often to help lower the fever.

- Give him carefully controlled doses of paracetamol for his fever if your doctor approves it and remember to use TCM (Traditional Chinese Medicine) during recuperation to help his liver recover.

- You can give him medications for nausea and vomiting.

- Check him every hour until the critical phase has passed.

- Reduce the risk of falls and injury and, thus, bruising and bleeding.

- If his platelet count is low, skip brushing his teeth to avoid gum bleeding.

- Distract him from blowing his nose hard or picking it.

- Acetaminophen overdoses are the leading cause of acute liver failure in the United States. Tylenol (active ingredient: acetaminophen) damages the liver. Children's dosages are particularly critical.

For Watchful Parents

- Here's a tip from pediatrician Dr. Richard Mata, who has treated thousand of kids with Dengue at at Panabo Polymedic Hospital, The Philippines.
- During hospital rounds, when I notice that the fever has subsided, I ask, "is the child playful again?"
- If the parent or ward nurse answers "No doc, he still sleeps all the time," I need to do a repeat CBC *immediately* because of the possibility of Dengue. Failure to do so may mean harm to the child. If you are a parent with a presently admitted child with fever, no matter what the doctor says of the diagnosis (including me) **always keep watch if your kid remains sleepy or weak and not playful when the fever is gone**. If you see that then, as a parent, **you have the right to request a repeat CBC** – just to be sure.

When Should Your Child Return To Hospital?

- Better to be safe than sorry if these symptoms appear:
- If his blood platelet count is under 80,000.
- If there's bleeding from the nose or gums – without any injury.
- If he looks or acts unwell, lethargic, or drowsy
- If he has difficulty breathing.
- If he's not eating or drinking normally or vomiting.
- If he has severe abdominal pain and giddiness.

While Your Child is in Hospital

Politely make sure that the hospital...

- Checks his platelet level and blood concentration **every day**.
- Monitors vital signs (pulse, blood pressure) every hour to detect potential Dengue complications described earlier in this book.
- is prepared to administer an intravenous drip if required. Ask a nurse.
- Is prepared to transfuse platelets or whole blood if the bleeding continues or if the platelet count is below 20,000 and falling.

When Can Your Child Go Home?

Hospitals will discharge kids who are well (talkative and playful) and have a rising platelet trend or platelet count above 70,000.

After he's discharged, take him back for a repeat blood test – which hospitals should recommend in his discharge letter – 1-2 weeks later to the hospital or your local GP to be absolutely sure that his platelet count is back to normal.

If he still feels very tired give him at least another week of rest at home.

Can Your Child Be Infected Again?

Yes. There are 4 strains of Dengue viruses. Infection with one strain provides temporary protection against only that particular strain. Future infection by other strains is possible and re-infection is extremely dangerous.

Can Your Child Spread Dengue To Others?

If a mosquito bites him while he's in the infectious phase, then that mosquito will spread the infection to the household and neighbors. But Dengue is not transmitted directly from one person to another, so it's fine for him to have as many visitors as he wishes.

Immunization?

There is currently no vaccine to protect against Dengue.

Preventing Infection

Severe Dengue usually develops in people who have already had Dengue. Having a Dengue infection doesn't make your child immune. It makes him more vulnerable. Prevention is vitally important.

The Centers for Disease Control and Prevention (CDC) suggests that using repellents containing DEET or picaridin (KBR 3023) usually provide longer-lasting protection than other repellents, and oil of lemon eucalyptus provides longer-lasting protection than other plant-based repellents. You can find these products in the 'Traps & Insecticides' chapter.

You can reduce his chances of his picking up Dengue by eliminating mosquitos at home, at school, and around his play areas. Old tires collect water where *Aedes* breed, as do rotting vegetation and containers as small as bottle-caps – especially in the monsoon season when humidity is high and stagnant water evaporates slowly. You can also:

- Dress him in light-colored, long-sleeved shirts and trousers to reduce exposed skin. Dark colors attract mosquitoes.

- Train him to rub on herbal mosquito repellents like lemon eucalyptus oil.

- Always use mosquito nets while he's sleeping.

- Install mosquito screens/meshes on all your doors and windows.

- Use air conditioning if mosquitos are numerous: it keeps them at bay.

- *Aedes* are active at dawn and dusk. Reserve these times for indoor activities.

- Use an appropriate repellent. Read the *Insecticides & Repellents* chapter before you rub anything on your kids' skin.

DEET is a dangerous neurotoxin that is approved for use on children with no age restriction. DEET is an effective mosquito repellent but many parents are concerned about its safety for children. The issue is still not settled but DEET is often the lesser of two evils: its toxicity is uncertain and probably insignificant if you do not use it long-term. But, if infection is likely, the real damage done by Dengue probably outweighs potential harm from DEET. So, if you're vacationing in a Dengue area, slap on the DEET every day following, of course, the guidelines below.

There is no restriction on the percentage of DEET in the product for use on children, since data do not show any difference in effects between young animals and adult animals in tests done for product registration. The EPA claims that there are no data showing incidents that suggests a need to restrict the use of DEET. The data referenced in the *Insecticides & Repellents* chapter may lead you to a different conclusion.

If you decide to use DEET on your child, here are some guidelines:

1. Avoid DEET for children <2 months of age.
2. For all other children use DEET concentration between 10% – 30%.
3. Do NOT use DEET with sunscreens. Sunscreens are often applied repeatedly because they can be washed off. DEET is not water-soluble and will last up to 8 hours. Repeated application increases the toxic effects of DEET.
4. Apply DEET sparingly on exposed skin; do not use it under clothing.
5. Do not use DEET on the hands of young children.
6. Avoid applying it to areas around the eyes and mouth.

7. Do not use DEET over cuts, wounds or irritated skin.

8. Wash treated skin with soap and water after returning indoors; wash treated clothing.

9. Avoid spraying in enclosed areas.

10. Do not use DEET near food.

11. If you suspect that your that your child is reacting to a repellent, stop using it, wash his skin, then call your local poison control center. In the USA, that's 1-800-222-1222. – The American Academy of Pediatrics

A higher concentration of DEET doesn't give you better protection is better - just that it will last longer. Repellents with 20% DEET last up to four hours, and one with 6.65% DEET lasts only two hours. Actual protection varies depending on conditions like temperature, perspiration and water exposure.

If you reapply the repellent regularly when you are together outdoors for long periods, or if your child will only be outside for a few hours, a repellent with 10% or less DEET should be enough. If you live in an infected area, rub on some low-strength DEET if your child will be outdoors during the peak mosquito feeding times, post-dawn and pre-dusk.

7. PREGNANCY & DENGUE

The number of women travelling during pregnancy combined with the geographical spread of Dengue means that more pregnant woman are contracting Dengue. Pregnancy doesn't increase the incidence of Dengue or its severity, and pregnant women experience the same progression of Dengue symptoms as everyone else. But Dengue infection *can* affect their later health and the health of their unborn babies, increasing the risks of

- Pre-eclampsia
  - thought to occur when the placenta doesn't work properly.
  - can have serious effects on both you and your baby if it is not promptly treated.
  - comes with high blood pressure, sudden swelling of your face, hands or feet.
  - sometimes accompanied by rapid weight gain.
  - usually happens in the second half of pregnancy, mostly in the third trimester.
  - affects the placenta and can impact your baby's growth by restricting the flow of oxygen and nutrients to him.
- Low birth weight
- Premature birth (pre-term labor)
- Caesarean birth
- Miscarriage

What precautions should I take?

1) If you're pregnant and traveling to, or living in, a Dengue-affected area take every precaution described in this book.

2) Reduce your use of DEET mosquito repellent by applying it to your clothing instead.

3) During earlier pregnancy consider Dengue a serious hazard and take extreme precautions.

4) Late-term, avoid travelling to Dengue-endemic areas.

5) **Tell your doctor you've been in a Dengue endemic area!** Your doctor may never have seen a case of Dengue and your symptoms may be atypical and confound diagnosis. Help her help you.

6) If you try it, be careful with your dosage of papaya leaf juice. Unconfirmed reports suggest that it may be unsafe for pregnant women.

Can I Transmit Dengue to my Baby?

Vertical transmission of the Dengue virus from the mother into the infant's bloodstream was described in 64.0% of women in case reports and and 12.6% of women in case series, as well as in one comparative study.

The authors (Pouliot, Xiong, et al.) conclude that there is a risk of vertical transmission but "whether maternal Dengue infection is a significant risk factor for adverse pregnancy outcomes is inconclusive". Stay tuned. You can read their entire report here...

Can I breastfeed my baby if I have Dengue?

Research suggests it might *be even better to breastfeed*. Breast milk can contain anti-Dengue antibodies that help protect your baby from Dengue infection.

What Do Scientists Say?

Case reports examined in a recent study showed high rates of

- cesarean deliveries (44.0%)

- pre-eclampsia (12.0%)

- preterm birth (16.1%) and

- cesarean delivery (20.4%).

- an increase in low birth weight among infants born to infected women. You can read the entire report here Maternal Dengue and Pregnancy Outcomes: a Systematic Review, by Pouliot, Xiong, et al.

Download a 1-Page Summary

Download Dengue and Pregnancy, from the Centers for Disease Control, here.

8. SEVERE DENGUE

Dealing with Dengue Hemorrhagic Fever (DHF)

The disease formerly known as 'Dengue hemorrhagic fever' (DHF) is now called *Severe Dengue*. In the past it's also been known as *Philippine*, *Thai,* or *Southeast Asian hemorrhagic fever* and *Dengue shock syndrome (DSS)*. It became visible in the 1950s during Dengue epidemics in Thailand and the Philippines.

Fast forward 60 years: severe Dengue affects most Asian and Latin American countries and is a leading cause of hospitalization and death among children in those regions. About 500,000 people with severe Dengue are hospitalized each year and it's a leading cause of serious illness and death among children in some Asian countries. In 2013, 2.35 million cases of Dengue were reported in the Americas alone, of which 37,687 cases were severe.

Reported cases of severe Dengue have been rising steadily in recent years, partly due to better public health awareness programs and improved diagnostic procedures.

About 500,000 people with Severe Dengue require hospitalization each year, many of them children. About 12,000 die. That means 1,000 people die every month from Severe Dengue. And the frequency of occurrence of the Severe form of Dengue is rising: it's reached 50% in some parts of Mexico.

With proper treatment the World Health Organization (WHO) estimates a mortality rate of 25 per 1,000 infections. Without proper treatment the mortality rate rises to 20%. Infants under 12 months of age are especially at risk of dying from DHF.

Several of my friends have had severe Dengue and all lived to tell the tale. One of them, Petra, tells her tale in this video. The trick is diagnosing it and treating it early. Treating it is a job for professionals, preferably in hospital. Here's a layman's guide to Severe Dengue:

Who's most at risk?

- Infants and children under 10. Most severe Dengue deaths occur in children.
- People who've had Dengue before.
- Females. Sorry, gals.
- People with a high body mass index.
- People carrying a high viral load.
- People with chronic diseases like diabetes and asthma.

What are the symptoms?

Since most Dengue first infections go unnoticed, it's safest to assume that *anyone* with Dengue has been infected before, and to watch for the following signs Here's the complete list. Everyone's experience will differ:

- Any or all the symptoms of 'normal' Dengue
- Temperature drops 3–7 days after symptoms began
- Bleeding (i.e., hemorrhaging) under the skin causing purple bruises
- Bleeding from the nose or gums, uterus
- Red eyes, throat
- Sore throat, cough, nausea, vomiting
- Impaired consciousness (like being drunk)
- Spitting up/vomiting blood
- Black, tarry stools (feces, excrement)
- Enlarged liver
- Swollen glands

- Low platelet count

- Heart problems (as severe as acute myocarditis)

- Low blood pressure leading to circulatory collapse. This is the "shock" part of Dengue
  Shock Syndrome: it occurs 2–6 days after symptoms appear: a sudden collapse, cool,
  clammy arms and legs (the trunk is often warm), weak pulse, and blue-tinged skin around
  the mouth.

- Rapid, weak pulse

- Drowsiness or irritability

- Abdominal pain

- Persistent vomiting

- Difficulty breathing

- Pneumonia.

- When the fever declines, a 24–48 hour period begins when the smallest blood vessels
  (capillaries) begin to leak, allowing the fluid component to escape from the blood vessels
  into your gut and lung cavities.

If you see any combination of those symptoms, GO IMMEDIATELY to an emergency room or
your closest health care provider!

The most visible symptom of severe Dengue is those leaking blood vessels: exactly what we *don't*
want them to do! Physicians call it *capillary permeability*: our capillaries allow the fluid and protein
in our blood to leak through their walls. Leaking capillaries are probably caused by our own
immune system's response, but researchers have yet to confirm that. The related symptom is
disordered blood clotting, which shows up as blood clots with no apparent external cause.

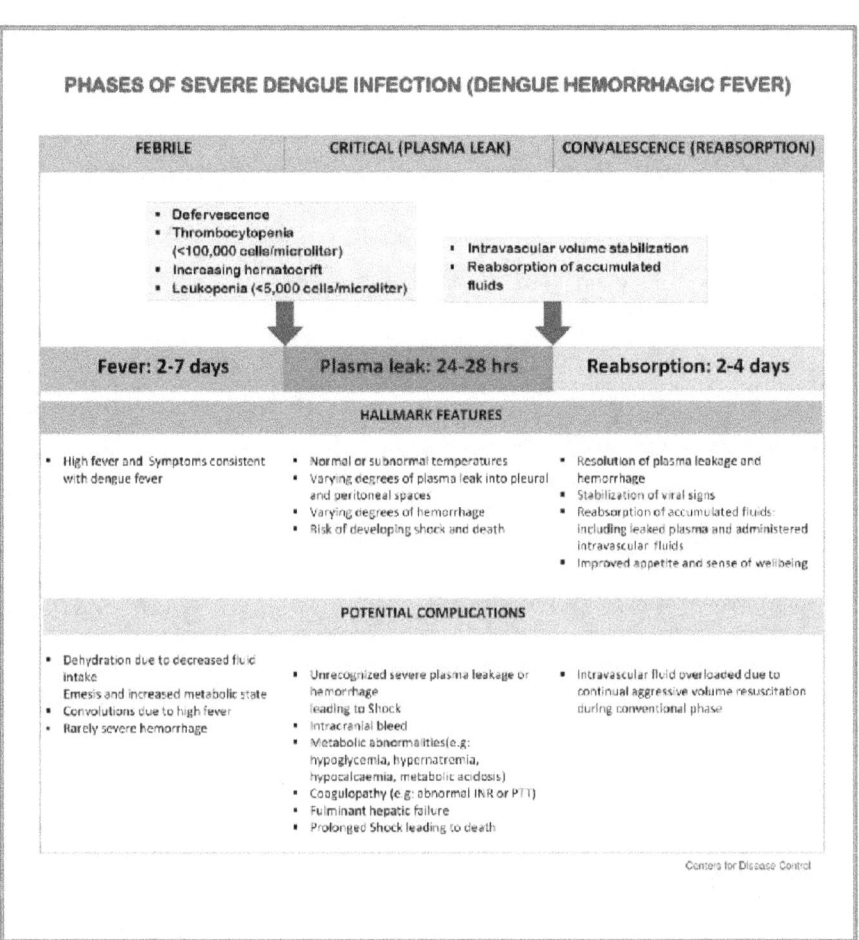

PHASES OF SEVERE DENGUE INFECTION (DENGUE HEMORRHAGIC FEVER)

FEBRILE	CRITICAL (PLASMA LEAK)	CONVALESCENCE (REABSORPTION)

• Defervescence
• Thrombocytopenia
  (<100,000 cells/microliter)
• Increasing hematocrift
• Leukopenia (<5,000 cells/microliter)
	• Intravascular volume stabilization
	• Reabsorption of accumulated
	  fluids	

Fever: 2-7 days	**Plasma leak: 24-28 hrs**	**Reabsorption: 2-4 days**

HALLMARK FEATURES

• High fever and Symptoms consistent with dengue fever	• Normal or subnormal temperatures • Varying degrees of plasma leak into pleural and peritoneal spaces • Varying degrees of hemorrhage • Risk of developing shock and death	• Resolution of plasma leakage and hemorrhage • Stabilization of viral signs • Reabsorption of accumulated fluids: including leaked plasma and administered intravascular fluids • Improved appetite and sense of wellbeing

POTENTIAL COMPLICATIONS

• Dehydration due to decreased fluid intake Emesis and increased metabolic state • Convolutions due to high fever • Rarely severe hemorrhage	• Unrecognized severe plasma leakage or hemorrhage leading to Shock • Intracranial bleed • Metabolic abnormalities(e.g: hypoglycemia, hypernatremia, hypocalcaemia, metabolic acidosis) • Coagulopathy (e.g: abnormal INR or PTT) • Fulminant hepatic failure • Prolonged Shock leading to death	• Intravascular fluid overloaded due to continual aggressive volume resuscitation during conventional phase

Centers for Disease Control

Treating Severe Dengue

Treating severe Dengue is a job for professionals. If your local professionals are unfamiliar with dengue, here's an excellent download for them prepared by the Centers for Disease Control. And here are some of the things your hospital will be doing in its intensive care unit:

- *Hourly monitoring* for the first few days. Shock may occur or recur suddenly (hence its former name: Dengue *shock* syndrome, or DSS).

31

- Platelet count and hematocrit levels taken and recorded serially because they indicate the *drop in platelets and rise in volume percentage of red blood cells* that indicate severe Dengue infection.
- Immediately replacing fluids when vascular collapse (shock) is indicated and, usually,
- Administering oxygen if blood oxygen drops.
- Giving blood transfusions if necessary to control bleeding.

And Here's What They'll Avoid When Treating Severe Dengue

- Administering aspirin or ibuprofens.
- Administering intravenous therapy before there's real evidence of hemorrhage and bleeding.
- Delaying blood transfusions unless hematocrit drops and there are clear signs of bleeding.
- Administering steroids. They don't help.

Recovery Signs

- Stable pulse, blood pressure and respiration
- Normal temperature
- Absence of external or internal bleeding
- Appetite returns
- No vomiting
- Healthy urine output
- Stable hematocrit

Possible Complications

Severe Dengue causes a wide range of complications depending on the patient's previous history and current health. Here's a list of them:

- Seizures

- Hypovolemic (decreased blood plasma volume) shock

- Acute mycarditis

- Hemophagocytic syndrome: increased capillary permeability and vasodilation can result in

  ○ ascites, pleural effusion, periorbital edema or

  ○ a rise in circulating hematocrit by 20+% due to loss of intravascular plasma volume.

- Liver dysfunction/injury in more than two thirds of cases.

- Right upper quadrant pain, hepatomegaly, and jaundice, reflecting liver cell injury induced by tissue ischemia and circulatory impairment.

- Fulminant hepatic failure – a consequence of the marked hepatocellular necrosis that follows circulatory collapse. Such patients may also have

  ○ disseminated intravascular coagulation and hemorrhage.

  ○ Acalculous cholecystitis associated with

  ○ fever,

  ○ right upper quadrant pain,

  ○ abnormal liver tests, and

  ○ a thickened gallbladder wall with absence of cholelithiasis at ultrasound.[15]

- Clinical pancreatitis (rare).

- Reye syndrome, acute parotitis

- Diarrhea associated with high fever.

- Residual brain damage.

- Death.

Read the complete report on Medscape.

9. PAINKILLERS & YOUR LIVER

The number of deaths involving commonly prescribed painkillers is higher than the number of deaths by overdose from heroin and cocaine combined. McGill University

Dengue fever may cause hepatic injury and transaminase elevation similar to that in patients with conventional viral hepatitis. In epidemic or endemic areas, Dengue fever infection should be considered in the differential diagnosis of hepatitis. – (NIH, NLM).

The first thing most people do when they get Dengue is reach for a painkiller which, while it provides immediate relief, brings its own set of liver problems. Here's why:

1. Dengue damages the liver of 30–60% of infected people.

2. *All* known painkillers – Acetaminophen, Ibuprofen, and Aspirin – cause liver damage.

3. Liver-damaging painkillers + liver-damaging Dengue = (possibly irreversible) liver damage.

Western medicine is great for stabilizing your vital signs but pays little attetnion to side-effects and after-effects. So how to minimize liver damage? TCM (Traditional Chinese Medicine) has been refining Dengue herbal formulae for 1200 years to help your liver recover, as you'll see in the next chapter.

About Pain Relievers

Acetaminophen overdoses are the leading cause of acute liver failure in the United States. Tylenol (active ingredient: acetaminophen) can damage your liver. 4 gm/day (12 regular-strength Tylenol tabs) is the upper limit, but that might be too much for some. Children's dosages, as I mentioned earlier, are particularly critical. Large doses are the main risk, but there are reports of people developing liver problems after taking small amounts of acetaminophen for long periods.

You may be taking more of it than you realize because acetaminophen is an ingredient in many OTC cold and headache medicines. People who drink alcohol regularly or have a less than healthy liver are more vulnerable to acetaminophen's toxic effects, so the safety threshold for them is lower. Heavy drinkers shouldn't take more than 2 grams daily.

NSAIDs <u>are leading causes of Drug-Induced Liver Injury (DILI)</u> : Most painkillers, like ibuprofen, naproxen and diclofenac (Cataflam, Voltaren), are nonsteroidal anti-inflammatory drugs (NSAIDs). Here are some aspects of NSAID use:

1. **All NSAIDs may increase heart attack risk**. NSAIDs revolutionized the treatment of pain but have the drawback of being hard on the stomach; *in extreme cases they cause gastrointestinal bleeding*. And, since Dengue *also* causes gastrointestinal bleeding, NSAIDs must be used with caution.

2. **Naproxen may be the safest painkiller if you have heart problems**. Of all the NSAIDs, naproxen seems to increase heart attack risk the least, but it has all the same risks for Dengue patients as the other NSAIDs.

3. **Low doses of Celebrex seem to be safe**. Despite the scandal (and 500,000 premature deaths from Vioxx and Bextra) Celebrex is still on the market, and at doses below 200 mg/day doesn't seem to increase the risk of heart attack.

4. **If NSAIDs bother your stomach** or you're at high risk for gastrointestinal complications, taking a proton pump inhibitor like omeprazole (Prilosec) or lansoprazole (Prevacid) can help. Talk to your physician.

5. **NSAIDs,** including the COX-2 drugs, tend to boost blood pressure, especially if have high blood pressure already and are taking medication to control it. Since blood pressure fluctuations can be dramatic and dangerous for Severe Dengue patients, these need to be used with great caution.

6. **NSAIDs,** including the COX-2 drugs, are hard on the kidneys and can cause kidney failure.

There is great individual variation in how people react to pain relievers. Your genes matter. The size of the dose matters. It may take some trial and error to find the pill that works best for you. You will only use painkillers for a few days so, unless you have a preexisting condition, you should be safe. Many risks associated with painkillers emerge only after long-term or heavy use.

For a complete discussion of painkillers, read this Harvard Medical School Family Guide.

10. RECOVERY & TCM

As I mentioned in the previous chapter, Western medicine is great for rescuing us in life-threatening situations but clueless about strengthening, tonifying, and re-balancing our systems once our vital signs stabilize. In fact, it's skeptical that such a thing is even possible. But since both Dengue and painkillers cause liver damage, our livers need help. Happily, that's where Eastern medicine complements Western techniques nicely.

When we hear the words "Traditional Chinese Medicine" (TCM) we think of acupuncture. But acupuncture is only a small part of Chinese medicine. 90% of TCM is devoted to diagnostics and herbal medicine. Most acupuncturists are not trained in Chinese herbal medicine, which takes much longer to master, and many herbal doctors are not trained in acupuncture.

The easiest way to find a TCM doctor trained in herbal medicine is to go to the nearest Chinese herb shop. They usually have a doctor in the back. He will tailor your prescription to your individual symptoms. Don't be put off by the informality of the scene. That's how Chinese like to operate because it keeps costs down– as you'll see when you pay your bill. Your TCM doctor will give you a series of prescriptions for each stage of your recovery. Remember to watch the pharmacist making up your prescription. It's a fascinating process and smells amazing.

You don't have to suffer Dengue after-effects for months or years if you use TCM. Tell your TCM doctor that you've had 骨痛热症 or 登革熱. If you have difficulty communicating, show her this page.

My TCM physician, Dr Boonrat, is the daughter of a TCM practitioner and is married to a TCM practitioner. They operate a beautiful clinic in the heart of Chiang Mai, Thailand, where they see patients from around the world. Dr. Boonrat is a noted diagnostician and is as happy chatting about platelet counts as about moxibustion. Since Dengue is endemic in Thailand she has treated hundreds of sufferers over her 30 years in practice. Here are her thoughts:

When I was young, I never got Dengue fever, nor did my brother, sister, mother or grandmother.

But my son got it – twice. The first time when he was in kindergarten, around four years old. My husband and I were away in Bangkok [Dr. Boonrat lives in Chiang Mai] for a conference and couldn't come back. His Auntie was looking after him and called us. We said, "Oh my God, such a high, high, high fever!

We couldn't leave the conference because we had to present at paper, so I called a good friend who's a physician at a local hospital. "Please go to my home! Please take care of my little Tan! What's wrong with him?" He went over to our house, called me and said, "I have to take your little one to hospital and administer an IV".

I said, "Okay, please take care, because we can't get back for 72 hours".

That was first time. Then around grade four he got another fever infection. Everyone was home this time. We didn't think he would get another infection. So we gave him some Chinese herbs and, unsure whether it was Dengue fever, we checked his platelet count, then figured out that it was another fever type. I don't remember which one, it was so long ago.

I suspected that this mosquito bite probably occurred at school and, when I checked with the school, they told me that one girl and two boys had already contracted Dengue. But the teacher doesn't know to isolate them and didn't inform the parents. And some of them has been diagnosed with severe hemorrhagic dengue and had to be hospitalized. From that point of view I think maybe we, Thailand or Chiang Mai, did not work well enough together about isolating such cases and doing prevention work.

I remember how I grew up in this country, which is how my parents and grandparents grew up. There wasn't much difference between the generations before Thailand's recent development. Back then Dengue was practically unheard of.

Maybe the mosquitos have evolved since then? Or perhaps it's the way the Health Department blows chemical sprays everywhere? I don't allow spraying around my clinic because, number one, we are operating. It's not healthy and, judging by the smell, I don't believe that the spray promotes good health or even prevents mosquitoes. I have a question mark around that. And the offspring of mosquitoes that survive that chemical spray are even more difficult to control.

The second thing is that I talked to my mom, who is now 90 years old, and she pointed out that the changing of the seasons is no longer clear. We don't have spring, we have summer and what we call the rainy season. It's not clear cut. Sometimes we get rain earlier and sometimes the rainy season extends longer, longer, longer and all that water is really good news for the mosquitos that carry the virus. So maybe the changing of the seasons impacts the mosquito cycle and, therefore, the virus, which is good for them but not for us. Unlike mosquitoes, humans have long lives and so are slow to adapt.

In Chinese medicine we say that our body is a small part of the universe. And our universe is changing quickly, but we don't know how to adapt because our lifestyles and the climate are so different.

Our generation was very healthy. My generation – I'm 56 right now – have had a good lifestyle since we were young. We ate on time, didn't smoke, didn't drink, didn't eat snack food. I've recently started to drink a little tea and stay up late because of my studies. But people today, if you look on the street, stay up late at night because we have electricity. So electricity has replaced the sunlight and people forget about the sun and moon, stay up late at night, get up after sunrise, many hours after sunrise and they drink something, they eat something, and their lifestyle leads to a weakness in their own systems and even prolongs recovery from illness, including from Dengue.

When you cannot adapt to the yin and yang of nature then what you call your immune system – which in Chinese we call our defensive chi – is weakened. This is another possible cause of the spread of dengue to more than 50 million people a year, right?

If we want adapt to these changes we need to plan an appropriate lifestyle. And lifestyle is what Chinese Medicine really understands and treats intelligently.

[Postscript: two years ago I noticed that my energy was rising and falling for no apparent reason and that I'd developed a craving for sugar, which made me sleepy and cranky. I consulted Dr. Boonrat who changed my diet and prescribed a simple exercise routine. My symptoms disappeared and have never recurred].

1. Dengue can leave you exhausted for weeks and, in some cases, years. Your experience will differ, of course:

2. At age 50, for every day you spent in bed allow 1 month of recuperation. Younger folks recover quicker.

3. Don't plan any strenuous activities until you're back to full health.

4. Schedule regular naps.

5. Eat a healthy, balanced diet.

6. Quit alcohol and nicotine until you're completely over it.

7. Don't be surprised if you feel tired and lethargic weeks after your 'recovery'.

8. You'll feel depressed or anxious. Like many infections, Dengue predisposes you to depression for physiological reasons. And anxiety – in the background even when we're healthy – moves to the foreground.

9. Go to bed 8 hours before dawn.

10. Get up at dawn and stay out as long as you can.

11. Get plenty of morning sunlight full on your face. If you're recuperating in winter, allow for the additional burden of SAD (Seasonal Affective Disorder).

12. Be active, even if it's gentle activity like swimming or walking.

13. Build your stamina steadily. No heroics.

14. Do NOT use stimulants or anti-depressants. They can make matters worse.

15. Hang in there and this, too, shall pass.

Depression

It's common to have depression for weeks or even months after any infection. Dengue is no different. Here are some key points about post-Dengue anxiety and depression from the International Journal of Psychiatry in Medicine and their correlation with symptom severity.

531 consecutive patients who met the WHO criteria for Dengue fever admitted to Mayo Hospital, Lahore, were administered the Hospital Anxiety and Depression Scale (HADS). In addition to the HADS, the severity of their symptoms, like headache, myalgias/arthralgias, fever, and retro/periorbital pain, was assessed on a 3-point scale (mild, moderate, and severe).

- 60% of the patients met the criteria for anxiety.
- 62.2% of them met criteria for depression.
- Severity of fever, headache, myalgias and arthralgias, and retro/periorbital pain was positively correlated with both anxiety and depression. – Read the complete article here

Hair Loss

Beginning about two months after the recovery stage, almost 45% of people notice some hair loss that lasts for 3-6 weeks. Don't freak out if your hairbrush is removing more hair than you'd like. The losses will end and, in most cases, your hair will grow back as beautiful as ever.

Relapses

Unlike malaria, Dengue fever doesn't have a liver stage that can lead to relapses. But you can become reinfected with a different strain of Dengue even if you have already had Dengue once. And reinfection puts you at greater risk of Severe Dengue.

11. DOCTORS & DRUGS

Prominent blogger Dr. Steven M. Fry describes himself as 'a scientist/handyman/teacher with bit of time on my hands' is married to a practicing scientist involved in Dengue research. They live in Mexico, where Dengue is endemic. For his lively discussions of Dengue, discussion, and fascinating case studies, start here, at yucalandia).

Dr. Fry has a scientist's eye for disease, not a clinician's, and his comments on clinicians (MDs) are sobering: Physicians, he points out,

- study very little science – especially compared to Chemists, Physicists, Molecular Biologists, and Biochemists – professionals who actually "do" science.

- don't learn critical thinking.

- don't learn how to do effective research.

- don't learn how to effectively *read* scientific research.

- don't typically *understand* scientific research because Medical Schools actively recruits people who are excellent at memorizing things – yet a good memory is a small component of being a good scientist.

- don't learn the statistics needed to determine if a research study has been well-designed or poorly-designed.

- for the past 30 years have been the THIRD LEADING CAUSE OF DEATH in the USA. Reliable, peer-reviewed, large studies of over 2 million patient records consistently show that Physician mis-diagnoses and Physician errors unnecessarily KILL 180,000 – 200,000 Americans every year. (These results do not include the harm and suffering caused by over-medication and physicians prescribing 10 – 30 different daily meds for old people – where the patient lives, but suffers unnecessarily – because the Physicians have NO IDEA of the interactions and side-effects of mixing meds).

- So if you're suffering from depression after a bout of Dengue (perfectly normal) DON'T BELIEVE what a typical physician tells you about depression. Physicians believe that brain-chemistry altering artificial drugs are the near-universal "cure" that is "required" for almost all cases of depression. But drugs are NOT the universal best answer.

- Consider that the current bible used by Physicians (the DSM) says that people who have the blues after the death of even an immediate family member are now CLINICALLY DEPRESSED ... and they should all be put on brain-altering drugs (serotonin uptake inhibitors).

Not good. Not good. And non-scientific.

Read more on Steve's blog, here.

12. IMMUNITY

In June, 2014, while researching this book I found an item on the WHO website: *There are four distinct, but closely related, serotypes of the virus that cause Dengue (DEN-1, DEN-2, DEN-3 and DEN-4). Recovery from infection by one provides lifelong immunity against that particular serotype.* I suspected that this was wrong but, not knowing how to contact the WHO, I contacted Dr. Fry using my *American Expat* address:

Dear Dr Fry, Your advice seems to differ from the WHO's take on immunity. You said: *Each Dengue infection confers a very brief immunity (3-4 months) to ONLY that strain of Dengue, but that single infection leaves the patient even more susceptible to more serious symptoms from the other 3 remaining Dengue strains (serotypes).* But the WHO says: *There are four distinct, but closely related, serotypes of the virus that cause Dengue (DEN-1, DEN-2, DEN-3 and DEN-4). Recovery from infection by one provides lifelong immunity against that particular serotype. However, cross-immunity to the other serotypes after recovery is only partial and temporary. Subsequent infections by other serotypes increase the risk of developing severe* Dengue. – W.H.O.

Am I missing something?

– American Expat in Chiang Mai

Dr. Fry responded:

Hi American Expat,

You are not missing anything. You have caught a grievous error by the programmers who typed the information into the WHO website. Oddly, the website you quote is written in British English – and that error directly contradicts the WHO's major hard-copy publications on Dengue.

It is very clear that prior Dengue infections DEFINITELY cause the patient to be MORE SUSCEPTIBLE to future Dengue Infections, and to HAVE WORSE SYMPTOMS with every subsequent Dengue infection due to sub-neutralizing antibodies created by the first Dengue infection.

THERE IS NO LIFETIME PROTECTION FROM DENGUE. So, please know that the W.H.O. DOES NOT say that a Dengue infection provides permanent protection. Just one FAULTY W.H.O. website makes this error.

Consider: *Both in vitro and in vivo, macrophages and monocytes participate in antibody-dependent enhancement (ADE) (18–20). ADE occurs when mononuclear phagocytes are infected through their Fc receptors by immune complexes that form between DENVs and non-neutralizing antibodies. these non-neutralizing antibodies result from previous heterotypic Dengue infections or from low concentrations of Dengue antibodies of maternal origin in infant sera (21)." from the official PEER REVIEWED – properly-edited W.H.O. publication.*

And the most recent research results, Nov. 2013, confirm that **any single Dengue infection can cause patients to be more susceptible to worse future Dengue infections**:

"Following natural Dengue virus (DENV) infection, humans produce some antibodies that recognize only the serotype of infection (type specific) and others that cross-react with all four serotypes (cross-reactive). Recent studies with human antibodies indicate that type-specific antibodies at high concentrations are often strongly neutralizing in vitro and protective in animal models. In general, cross-reactive antibodies are poorly neutralizing and can enhance the ability of DENV to infect Fc receptor-bearing cells under some conditions. Type-specific antibodies at low concentrations also may enhance infection. –

WHO's web programmers need better oversight/editing,

All the best, Steve.

The moral of this tale is that, in serious matters like Dengue, double-check the information I'm

giving you here and check advice from your physicians, your friends, and even the W.H.O.

Instead of a Dengue infection granting you life-long immunity it makes you *more* susceptible to *worse* infections, the symptoms worsen and the possibility of death increases dramatically with each subsequent infection. A single infection leaves you even more susceptible to more serious symptoms from the three remaining Dengue strains (*serotypes*). That's why it's useful to understand how reinfected people often develop the severe form:

- The Dengue virus has 4 distinct, closely related, serotypes: different strains of Dengue virus that are 60-80% similar with only subtle differences in their surface proteins: DEN-1, DEN-2, DEN-3 and DEN-4.

- Re-infection by the first strain is possible after 4 months. Infection by the other 3 strains is possible in the meantime.

- Recovery from infection by one serotype provides only temporary immunity against that particular serotype.

- That immune response produces specific antibodies to that subtype's surface proteins that prevents the virus from binding to your macrophage cells (the target cell that Dengue viruses infect) and gaining entry.

- However, if *another* subtype of Dengue virus infects you, the virus will activate your immune system to *attack it as if it was the first subtype*.

- Your immune system is tricked because the 4 subtypes have very similar surface antigens.

- So the antibodies bind to the surface proteins but do not inactivate the virus.

- Your immune response attracts numerous macrophages, which the virus infects because it has not been inactivated. This is called Antibody-Dependent Enhancement (ADE) of a viral infection.

- This makes the viral infection much more acute. The body releases cytokines that cause the endothelial tissue to become permeable, resulting in hemorrhagic fever and fluid loss from the blood vessels.

- All forms of Dengue fever are associated with the same four viruses. So if your neighbor develops a mild infection do not assume that you or your children will have the same form of the disease – even if you're bitten by the same mosquito.

- There is a possible long-term beneficial effect: people who live in areas where Dengue is endemic seem to have unusual resistance to similar flaviviruses like West Nile Virus, Saint Louis Encephalitis, Dengue, and Cache Virus.

To stay current on this discussion visit Steve's blog.

13. LAB TESTS

If you suspect Dengue request an (inexpensive) Complete Blood Count (CBC) including platelets. Here's a rough guide to the results:

- If you've got Dengue you'll see an elevated HCT (hematocrit, or packed cell volume) along with a depressed platelet count.

- If your platelet count is below 100,000 it's probably Dengue and you're in danger of developing severe Dengue. Go to hospital.

- If your white blood count is elevated you probably have a bacterial infection and need immediate medical attention and possibly hospitalization.

- If you've got Dengue your white blood count will be normal or low.

Serology Tests

If your hospital wants to identify your strain of Dengue they'll order serology tests. They're especially valuable because they help public health authorities track infectious strains accurately. With the exception of serology, *these tests have diagnostic value only during the acute phase* of the illness. Each test requires a page-long description, which is outside the scope of this book. If your doctor wants to order tests, here are the ones she'll be considering:

- Virus isolation

- Nucleic acid detection

- RT-PCR

- Real-time RT-PCR

- Isothermal amplification methods

- Detection of antigens

- Serological tests

- MAC-ELISA

- IgM/IgG ratio

- IgA

- Haemagglutination-inhibition test

- Haematological tests

Timing

Timing is everything with Dengue tests. The window of opportunity for administering the NS-1 test and platelet count is days 1–4 after onset of fever/symptoms. If this is your first infection and your doctor suspects complications, get tested between Days 4-7 for Severe Dengue (DHF or DSS) symptoms.

Some commonly-used lab tests do not detect Dengue in people with a prior Dengue infection until Day 10 after onset of symptoms, because prior Dengue infections heavily interfere with the patient's immune response to the new infection. Read more (Yucalandia). So patients should be watched carefully for symptoms of bleeding, shock or abdominal symptoms during this period. The chart below is a useful indicator:

When tests become positive

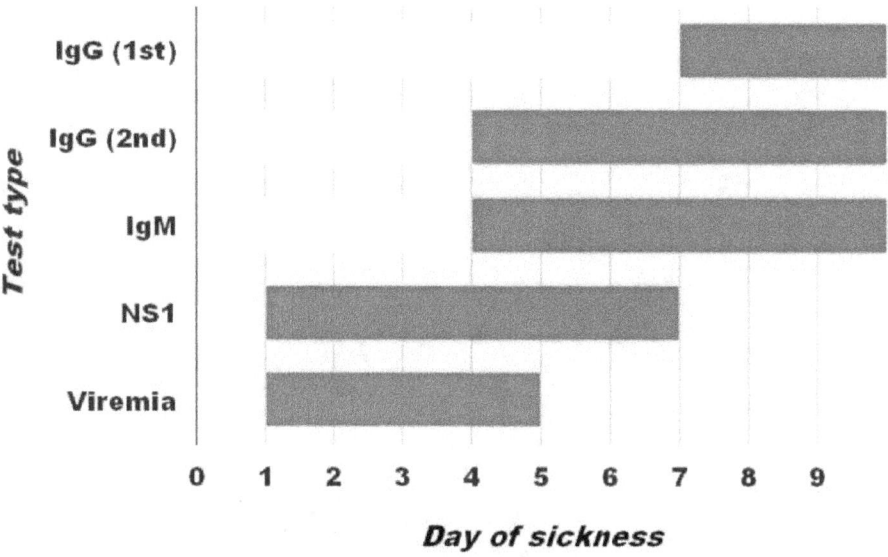

'Day zero' is the onset of symptoms. '(1st)' refers to primary infections and '(2nd)' refers to those with secondary infections. – Diagram by James Heilman, MD. Creative Commons Licence.

14. SOMEBODY STOP ME!

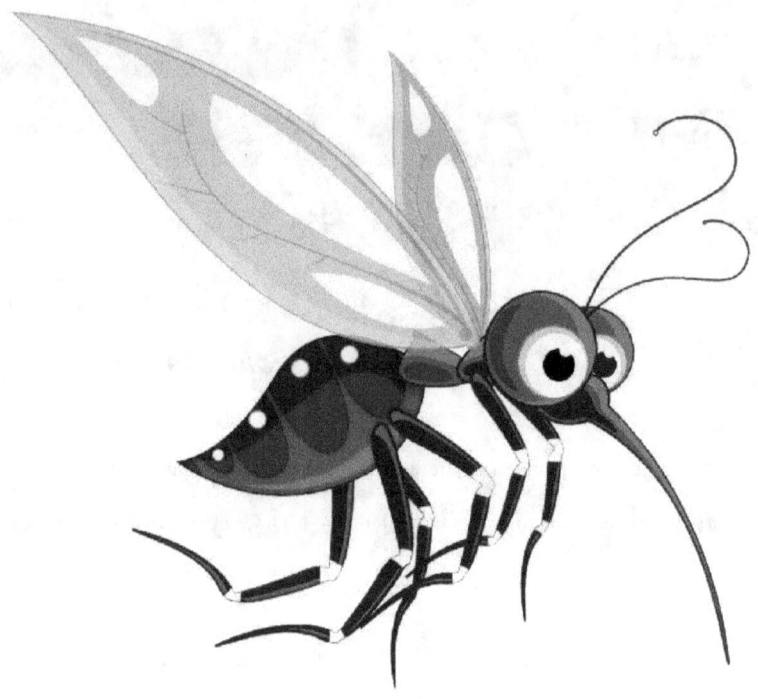

Though my family name, *Aegypti*, means 'Egyptian', we're originally from Southern China. We don't think of ourselves as Egyptian *or* Chinese, of course. My ancestors pioneered world travel in the early 1200s and we've been urbanized, sun-loving global citizens ever since. I myself was hatched near Jupiter Beach, Florida.

Aedes, in case you're wondering, means 'household': we're indoor folks like you. We enjoy human company (we're *anthroprophiles*) so much we've become dependent on you. Our wild cousins rarely live more than a month but, if you provide our simple needs, we can live for 6 months in your house.

You're reading this because at some point a wild mosquito cousin of mine accidentally inoculated one of your human ancestors with a flavivirus called *Dengue*. One of my indoor ancestors unsuspectingly got a dose of the virus while snacking on your ancestor. It had no effect on my ancestor but, unfortunately, it has nasty effects on yours.

Since that fateful day, whenever one of us gets Dengue virus from one of you – and that's the only way we <u>can</u> get it – we can't help transmitting it for months, every time we snack on you.

In the tropics my eggs need only a week in a teaspoon of water to grow up. Almost any water will do in. Abandoned swimming pools are great of course, but old tires and flower pots are fine too. Piles of junk are perfect because they provide cool, dark, moist crannies. My broods have hatched in bowls, earthenware jars, tin cans, vases, cups, bottles and bottle caps, plates, pots and pans.

It's my secret dream to have a thousand healthy children around me when my time comes to pass on. Unfortunately, one meal of your blood only provides enough nutrition for me to lay a single batch of eggs, and I've laid many batches in my lifetime.

So each egg batch requires a new blood meal, which is what leads to diseases being transmitted amongst you humans: if I bite you and you're infected, then I get infected, too. When it's time for me to lay more eggs the odds are that I'll bite someone who's *not* infected.

Then I'll be the villainess and people will start reaching for their spray cans. Sometimes I feel victimized.

15. CALL ME AEDES

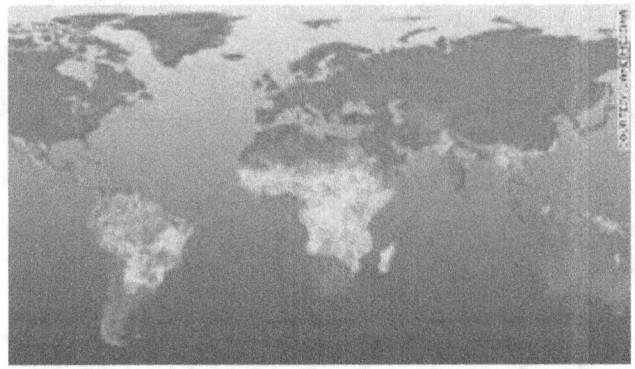

The disease burden has risen from 15,000 cases per year in the 1960s to 390 million today – more than half the population of Europe. Once seen as an urban and peri-urban disease, Dengue is increasingly becoming a challenge in rural areas as well. – Red Cross.

Mosquitoes are the most dangerous animals on earth. The little beggars have <u>killed more people</u> than all the wars in history. While snakes and sharks would prefer to avoid us, mosquitoes find us irresistible.

Fifty years ago, Dengue was established in only nine countries. Now it's in 100. Mosquitoes are spreading more and more disease – and there's more of it to spread because infected people from places where Dengue flourishes are visiting temperate areas, which are themsleves warming and experiencing new rainfall patterns.

Increased global warming along with extended rain patterns mean that Dengue-carrying mosquitos are spreading north and south into states that never thought they'd have to deal with such an exotic tropical disease. Global temperature increases speed immature mosquito development, virus development, and mosquito biting rates – which increases contact with humans. Know the enemy:

- Aedes is distributed around the globe between latitudes 35° N – 35° S. They've been found as far north as 45° N in summer but haven't survived the winters. Aedes is relatively uncommon above 1000 meters altitude (3,300 ft) because of lower temperatures.
- Aedes is one of the most efficient vectors for arboviruses like Dengue Virus because it usually bites several times before completing its egg cycle and thrives in proximity to humans.
- Once Aedes' eggs are laid, they typically take 7 days to hatch and develop into adult mosquitoes.
- Dengue infected Aedes can live in the wild for 30 days and in your home for 6 months.
- Within the mosquito, the virus infects the mid-gut and subsequently spreads to the salivary glands over a period of 8-12 days.
- After virus incubation for 4–10 days, infected mosquitoes are capable of transmitting the virus for the rest of their lives.
- Aedes mosquitoes can fly very fast, unlike other mosquitos, and they inject an anesthetic with their saliva so you don't feel the bite.
- Typically, Aedes remain within 100 metres of where they hatch. They feed almost entirely on humans, mainly during daylight hours, both indoors and outdoors.
- Aedes that feed on human blood have better health and produce more offspring than their sisters that feed on other kinds of animal blood, though the reason for this is unknown.
- Aedes bite multiple people during each feeding period.
- You'll find Aedes' immature stages mostly in artificial water containers closely associated with humans – often indoors.
- Most female Aedes spend their lifetime – 6 months – in or around the houses where they emerge as adults.

- Dengue cannot be spread from person to person. People, not mosquitoes, move the virus rapidly within and between communities.

- Aedes tend to feed in the morning and the evening. They typically bite people's feet, ankles, and lower legs.

- Aedes are silent flyers and do not feed late at night. Mosquitoes that bother you late at night are not Aedes.

- Aedes eggs can withstand very dry conditions and remain viable for many months in the absence of water.

Epidemiology

"Dengue has been present for centuries. The first recorded symptoms compatible with Dengue were noted in a Chinese medical encyclopedia in 992 AD, originally published by the Chin Dynasty centuries earlier (265–420 AD), prior to being formally edited.

The disease was referred to as 'water poison' and was associated with flying insects. Epidemics that resembled Dengue, with similar disease course and spread, occurred as early as 1635 and 1699 in the West Indies and Central America, respectively. A major epidemic occurred in Philadelphia in 1780 and epidemics then became common in the USA into the early 20th century, the last outbreak occurring in 1945 in New Orleans. The viral etiology and the transmission by mosquitoes were only finally determined in the 20th century.

The origin of the primary mosquito vector, *Aedes aegypti,* is debated to be from either Africa or Asia. Regardless, by 1800 it was widespread throughout urban tropical coastal cities of the world due to the use of shipping vessels with commercial expansion. These shipping vessels allowed transportation of breeding sites for the vector along with humans to complete the transmission cycle, allowing for slow but evident introduction of the virus and the mosquito to coastal destinations around the world.

Epidemics were spaced by 10-40 year intervals due to this shipping mode of transport. Expansion of the disease heightened during World War II when troops began to disperse inland and utilize modern transportation within and between countries; thus epidemic Dengue became more far-reaching. By the end of the war transportation and rapid urbanization led to increased transmission of Dengue and hyperendemicity (multiple serotypes present) in most South East Asian countries, with subsequent emergence of the severe forms of Dengue.

Following WWII, Dengue epidemics appeared to be under control in Central and South America. The elimination of *Aedes* due to collaborative efforts with the yellow fever disease control campaign initiated by the Pan American Health Organization (PAHO), effectively restricted the transmission of Dengue throughout the American continent.

The lull in Dengue epidemics in the Americas was short-lived as the control campaign was discontinued in the 1970s. By the 1980s incidence had increased, and by 1995 pre-campaign levels were present in the Americas. Geographic expansion of epidemic Dengue from South East Asia in the late 20th century saw regions in the Pacific and Americas escalate from being non-endemic with no Dengue serotypes circulating, to hypo-endemic (one serotype present), and some hyper-endemic. Global Dengue incidence has increased precipitously over the last five decades and severe Dengue cases have also expanded. Prior to 1970, only nine countries had experienced severe Dengue cases, a number which has since quadrupled..." – Murray, Quam, Wilder-Smith: Epidemiology of Dengue: Past, Present and Future Prospects.

Some Epidemiology Links

Here are some useful facts and links. For more detail, click on the reference numbers, like [6], after each:

- Like most arboviruses, Dengue virus is maintained in nature in cycles that involve preferred blood-sucking vectors and vertebrate hosts.[6]

- The viruses are maintained in the forests of Southeast Asia and Africa by transmission from female Aedes mosquitoes to her offspring and to lower primates.[6]

- In towns and cities, the virus is primarily transmitted by the highly domesticated *Aedes aegypti*. In rural settings the virus is transmitted to humans by *A. aegypti* and other species of *Aedes* such as Aedes albopictus.[6]

- Due to a process called amplification, in all settings the infected lower primates or humans greatly increase the number of circulating Dengue viruses.[6]

- Dengue is endemic in more than 110 countries.

- It infects up to 500 million people worldwide a year, leading to half a million hospitalizations,[2][3] and approximately 25,000 deaths.[8]

- Dengue is reported in at least 22 countries in Africa but is likely present in all of them with 20% of the population at risk.[41]

- Dengue infection rates among people who have not been previously exposed to the virus, commonly 40% to 50% during epidemics, may reach 90%.

- Infections are most commonly acquired in the urban environment.[6] In recent decades, the expansion of villages, towns and cities in endemic areas, and the increased mobility of people has increased the number of epidemics and circulating viruses.

- Not only is the number of cases increasing as the disease spreads to new areas, but explosive outbreaks are occurring.

- Dengue fever, which was once confined to Southeast Asia, might now pose a threat to Europe.[5]

- Local transmission of Dengue was reported for the first time in France and Croatia in 2010 and imported cases were detected in three other European countries.

- In 2012, an outbreak of Dengue on Madeira islands of Portugal resulted in over 2,000 cases and imported cases were detected in 10 other countries in Europe apart from mainland

Portugal.

- In 2013, cases occurred in Florida (USA) and Yunnan Province, China.
- Dengue continues to affect several south American countries notably Honduras, Costa Rica and Mexico.
- Cuba, which had eradicated Dengue, has reported a new epidemic.
- In Asia, Singapore has reported an increase in cases after a lapse of several years and outbreaks have also been reported in Laos.
- In 2014, trends indicate increases in the number of cases in the Cook Islands, Malaysia, Fiji and Vanuatu, with Dengue Type 3 (DEN 3) affecting the Pacific Island countries after a lapse of over 10 years.
- The geographical distribution is around the equator with 70% of the total 2.5 billion people living in endemic areas from Asia and the Pacific.[42]
- Dengue is second only to malaria as a diagnosed cause of fever among returning travelers. [11]
- It is the most common viral disease transmitted by arthropods,[15] and has a disease burden (the impact of a health problem as measured by financial cost, mortality, morbidity, or other indicators) estimated at 1,600 disability-adjusted life years per million population.[16]

Read more here...

16. 99% PREVENTION

Five of my yoga-teacher friends share a house in Chiang Mai all got infected within two weeks of each other.

Neil, the first victim, got bitten by an infected mosquito at an outdoor beer garden where he was watching the Thai sun set. He slept in his un-netted bed. An *Aedes* mosquito living in the house bit him, became infected then bit Deirdre, whose bedroom is across the hall. Nobody had experience with Dengue so they allowed a mini-plague to break out in their home. Even the nurse who came to care for them became infected.

90% of *Aedes* mosquitoes collected in the homes of Dengue patients are infected with Dengue. Everyone near a Dengue patient risks contracting it, too.

Risk Reduction

You can reduce your chances of Dengue infection by 99% with a few simple precautions:

- If you have a Dengue patient in your house or neighborhood protect them and yourself from mosquitoes at all costs! Dengue-infected people can transmit their infection via Aedes for up to 2 weeks after their first symptoms appear. Your entire household can be infected in days.

- QUARANTINE THE INFECTED PERSON WITH MOSQUITO NETS, SPRAY THE ENTIRE HOUSE, AND TAKE SPECIAL PRECAUTIONS WITH NEIGHBORING CHILDREN.

- Completely eradicate mosquitoes from your home. I close all the windows and doors in one room, spray it thoroughly with Baygon, then move to the next room and repeat until I've treated every room. Then I close the house tight and go out for coffee. (An iced caramel latte frappe with whipped cream helps mask the smell of inscticide).

- Aedes lives, rests, and digests blood meals in cool, dark places, like under the bed and, attracted by our smell on our clothes, in clothes closets. I concentrate my mosquito spraying efforts on low, cool, dark places.

- Exclude mosquitoes from your living areas using tight window and door screens.

- Switch your 'mosquito consciousness' to daytime. Aedes activity peaks after sunrise and before sunset.

- Keep your lower legs, ankles, and feet covered. Wear long pants and socks.

- Patronize places with well-maintained insect screens. Remember, Aedes is as happy indoors as out. Indoors, you're a sitting duck for those speedy, silent, painless mosquitoes.

- Use fans wherever you go. Mosquitoes are easily blown away, so request a fan at restaurants, for example.

- No fan? Sit with your feet off the floor. Practice your Lotus posture.

- Choose locations away from mosquito breeding sites: no standing water unless it also has little fish that you can see. I have often been reassured that a lotus vase (always filled with water) has 'feesh' that will eat any mosquito larvae. I suggest you check the veracity of such claims.

- Move up. There are no mosquitos above the 6th floor, and few Aedes above the 2nd floor.

- Buy bottles, tubes, and cans of mosquito repellent. Keep the smallest in your pocket, one in the car, and one by the door and apply it to your exposed lower limbs before you leave the house in the morning. I keep a spray can of SC Johnson's OFF Active by my door. It's easy to apply and smells good. I wash it off as soon as I return.

- If used with a sunscreen, the CDC recommends applying the sunscreen before the repellent. If you're concerned about DEET – and you should be –see the chapter on Insecticides and Repellents.

- Outdoors, *Aedes* can breed in as little as a teaspoon of residual rainwater so the best way to eliminate Dengue and *Aedes* is to eliminate their breeding grounds. Get rid of anything around your property that collects standing water: old tires, pets' water bowls, old crockery, plastic rubbish, brush piles, etc., and drill holes in the bottom of flower pots and containers.

Rather than relying on weekly applications of chlorine or ammonia, cover unused toilets and drains with Saran wrap; it permanently blocks mosquitoes whereas chemicals dissipate over time.

Several fish species will help eliminate mosquitoes from larger water containers, open freshwater wells, irrigation ditches and industrial tanks. Guppies, Gambusia and Mollies breed fast and eat mosquito larvae.

Prevention in Singapore

Singapore is 80 miles from the equator and *really* tropical! I visit often, partly because it's the best-run country on earth. Singaporeans are the healthiest, longest-lived people in the tropics. Their public health department is powerful, expert, and extremely effective. Here's what 60 years' experience has led them to recommend:

- The best prevention is getting rid of mosquito breeding places.
- Change water in vases/ bowls, flowerpot plates, pet water containers on alternate days.
- Turn over all water storage containers and cover bamboo pole holders when not in use.
- Cover rarely used gully traps.
- Add prescribed amount of Temephos (trade name Abate) – an organophosphate larvicide used to treat water in roof gutters – at least once a month.
- Cover toilet bowls and floor traps when away from home for a few days.
- Fit all floor traps with anti-mosquito valves.
- Use air conditioning or windows/doors with mosquito screens to reduce the risk of being bitten by mosquitoes.

- Using mosquito repellents containing DEET as the active ingredient on exposed skin and clothing can also decrease the risk of being bitten by mosquitoes. But this method is not nearly as effective as environmental control.

17. INSECTICIDES & REPELLENTS

Most products will do the job if you're only going to be outside for a couple of hours, but for longer expeditions you'll need something that can give you up to 7 hours protection.

DEET is the most effective repellent in the human armory right now. It's a powerful synthetic neurotoxin and a powerful money-earner for many corporations. (It also dissolves plastics!). There is evidence that it can be dangerous, especially to children, and especially when used in conjunction with common sunscreens. If this concerns you, try some of the alternatives described below. And if you want to know more about natural pesticides there's no better place to start than the blog, Beyond Pesticides.

Natural Strategies

The combination of prevention and repulsion, though it requires effort, is healthiest for everyone and, especially, for children and pets. Here are some natural tricks of the trade:

- Eat raw garlic, cook with onion and bell pepper, and take vitamin B. All these foods help produce a body odor that mosquitoes find unattractive.
- Grow mint, roses, tuberose (*Polianthes tuberosa*), orchid tree (*Aglaia odorata var. microphylla*), and marigold. All repel mosquitoes to some degree.
- Burn the leaves of the lemon-scented gum eucalyptus (*Eucalyptus citriodora Hook*) for household protection.
- Use outdoor LED lights on your porch and around your house. They don't attract pests like other lights.

- Burn citronella candles outside.

The natural options are not available to everyone so mosquito sprays can be a good alternative. Some of the least toxic sprays include:

- **Oil of Lemon Eucalyptus** has been used for many years in China as a mosquito repellent. The Centers for Disease Control (CDC) recommends lemon eucalyptus oil repellents as a good alternative to DEET. The lemon eucalyptus oil's scent masks the lactic acid, ammonia, carbon dioxide, octenol, phenols, temperature, and humidity that cue mosquitoes to human presence, making it harder for mosquitoes to find us. According to CDC, this plant-based mosquito repellent provides protection time similar to 10% concentration DEET products. (Repel Lemon Eucalyptus Insect Repellent).

- **Essential Oils** – Some essential oils used in repellents include Cedarwood, Soybean Oil (www.biteblocker.com), and Geraniol (MosquitoGuard- www.wildroots.com, Bite Stop- www.bitestop.com, Bugband- www.bugband.net). Compared to products like Citronella, Geraniol proved effective. Against products containing 10% Deet, Geraniol also proved effective.

- **Picaridin** – a synthetic dervived from pepper. The CDC says its protection is comparable to DEET at similar concentrations (Cutter Advanced). It appears to have low potential for toxicity.

- **Citronella** – The active ingredient in those candles. It's in some natural spray blends like Insect Shield (Bug Off) Synergy: an undiluted, therapeutic grade blend of the essential oils of Citronella, Eucalyptus, Cedarwood, Lemongrass, Lavender, Litsea, Tea Tree, Patchouli & Catnip. If it doesn't repel your local mosquitoes you can always try it as a salad dressing.

Some Commercial Products

All these repellents have different durations of effectiveness so be sure to reapply them following the directions on the label to repel mosquitoes most effectively.

Product Name & Link: <u>**Cutter Lemon Eucalyptus Insect Repellent Pump Spray, 4-Ounce**</u>.

Sales Pitch: Cutter lemon eucalyptus pump spray is an effective, naturally plant to based repellent that repels mosquitoes for up to 6 hours. Contains oil of lemon eucalyptus to the only plant to based ingredient recommended by the centers for disease control and prevention (CDC).

Typical Review: Cutter Lemon Eucalyptus insect repellent is one of my favorite summer products for many reasons; it's made with clean, woodsy-scented natural lemon eucalyptus, one of the least offensive smelling repellent sprays around; it is non-greasy and clear, absorbing right into your skin; and best of all, it REALLY WORKS at repelling all flying summer bugs including mosquitoes, flies & gnats. I am an outdoor early a.m. gardener, so besides spraying exposed skin, I lightly spray my clothes with this product and there is never a stain and barely the mildest scent. The pump style bottle has great control, it releases according to your touch, so you can pump a light amount directly onto your skin, or a harder pump will release more into your palm for hand-to-body application. This bottle is also perfect when empty for make-your-own repellent, you can buy lemon eucalyptus oil here on Amazon, pour the vial into the bottle, add olive or baby oil as a mixer, and you have another effective all-natural insect repellent.

Average Score: 4.2/5

Product Name & Link: <u>**Bite Blocker Organic Insect Repellent Spray, 6 Oz**</u>.

Sales Pitch: Bite Blocker's proven effective Insect Repellent now in a highly effective waterproof formulation though enough for extreme environments and safe for the entire family. This Xtreme botanical formula provides protection form bites for up to 8 hours against mosquitoes, blackflies and more than 2 hours for ticks.

Typical Review: On a recent backpacking trip to the High Sierras, this stuff was a lifesaver (or should i say "tripsaver")! Where DEET failed, BiteBlocker passed-in flying colors! Yeah, the smell may be a little funky but who cares (at least it's from something natural and not some man-made "chemical"). Look, all i know is the mosquitoes are gone (right along with Mr. Miserable, Mr. Annoying and Mr. Painful). Thx Xtreme Sportsman, for making an all natural, human friendly, mosquito deadly product...that actually helps keep an enjoyable trip...enjoyable!!!

Average Score: 4.1/5.0

About DEET

DEET is a good chemical for protection against insects, but prolonged exposure results in neurological damage, and this is enhanced by other chemicals and medications. – Bahie Abou-Donia of the Duke University Medical Center.

There's no doubt that DEET is an effective insect repellent but its use has become highly controversial, with seizures reported among children.

Our regulatory bodies are less and less inclined to demand tests and product recalls. Even though the EPA claims that there is not enough information to implicate DEET in these incidents, in the interest of self-protection, familiarize yourself with DEET before you slap it on.

DEET is quickly absorbed through the skin and has caused adverse effects including large blisters and burning sensations. Laboratory studies have found that DEET can cause neurological damage, including brain damage in children.

What Lab Tests Say About DEET

Duke Medical University pharmacologist Mohamed Abou-Donia, Ph.D., who I quoted above, conducted numerous studies in rats which clearly demonstrated that

- Frequent and prolonged applications of DEET cause neurons to die in regions of the brain that control muscle movement, learning, memory and concentration.

- Rats treated with an average human dose of DEET (40 mg/kg body weight) performed far worse than control rats when challenged with physical tasks requiring muscle control, strength and coordination.

- With heavy exposure to DEET and other insecticides, humans may experience memory loss, headache, weakness, fatigue, muscle and joint pain, tremors and shortness of breath.

- There are even greater impacts when DEET exposure occurs in combination with pharmaceuticals and other pesticides, including permethrin, an insecticide commonly used for public mosquito control.

- According to Dr. Abou-Donia,

- Never use insect repellents on infants, and beware of using them on children in general.

- Never combine insecticides with each other or use them with other medications.

- Even an antihistamine could interact with DEET to cause toxic side effects.

- Until we have more data on potential interactions in humans, safe is better than sorry.

Do not use DEET in combination with sunscreens. Repeated application may increase the potential toxic effects of DEET and increase absorption rates and toxic effects by 300%. For more, read Drug Metabolism and Disposition.

Do not use DEET at concentrations above 30% – the Canadian regulatory limit. Based on lab results it's unwise to use United States formulations with DEET concentrations up to 100%.

For more information on alternatives to DEET see Beyond Pesticides mosquito and insect-borne diseases webpage.

How DEET Works

DEET (N,N-diethyl-3-methylbenzamide), slows or halts the actions of the enzyme acetylcholinesterase in both insects and mammals. This enzyme is typically found between nerve and muscle cells breaking down a messenger molecule after it has passed information from one cell to another. If the messenger isn't properly recycled it can build up and lead to paralysis. – Science News

---

Children and DEET

See the *Children & Dengue* chapter.

Current US Department of Defense Insect Repellent System:

The Defense Department is responsible for the health of 1 million employees who rotate through the tropics every year. Here's what the DOD's come up with:

1. Wear permethrin treated uniforms. If not using uniforms pre-treated by the manufacturer with permethrin, treat uniforms (except for Nomex uniforms such as flight suits) with permethrin clothing repellent and allow them to dry BEFORE putting them on. Do not treat pre-treated uniforms. Two self-treatment options are available. The first option is to use the Impregnation Kit (NSN 6840-01-345-0237) to treat one uniform. The treatment lasts for the life of the uniform (at least 50 washes). The second option is to use the aerosol can of permethrin (NSN 6840-01-278-1336). Each can treats one uniform, and the treatment lasts through 5-6 washes.

2. Wear uniform properly. Roll down shirt sleeves. Tuck pants into boots with the blousing

cords drawn tight. Tuck undershirt into pants. These measures will help protect the skin from biting insects (such as sand flies).

3. Apply DEET to exposed skin. Apply a thin coat of long-lasting DEET insect repellent lotion (NSN 6840-01-284-3982) to all EXPOSED skin. One application lasts for up to 12 hours, depending on the climate and how much you perspire. Follow all label directions.

4. The DOD, which in today's military must consider the needs of families with children, has this to say about DEET safety:

Q: Is there any reason I or others, including my family, shouldn't use DEET?

A: There is no reason one shouldn't use DEET unless one has a documented allergy to DEET or to other ingredients in the product. According to the American Academy of Pediatrics, products containing 30% or less DEET can be used safely on children greater than 2 months old (consult your pediatrician first). Apply it sparingly to children and don't apply it to their hands, which they often place in their eyes and mouths.

Q: Can I use an insect repellent containing DEET and sunscreen at the same time?

A: Yes. DEET can be used with sunscreen, but it may reduce the effectiveness of the sunscreen. To minimize this effect, apply sunscreen approximately 30 minutes to 1 hour prior to applying the DEET, so that the sunscreen has time to penetrate and bind to the skin. Sunscreen does NOT reduce the effectiveness of the DEET. Always use a sunscreen with an SPF appropriate for your skin type, whether or not using DEET.

Note: DEET should not be allowed to contact synthetic materials as it may discolor and eventually deteriorate these materials. Permethrin is safe on all fabrics except Nomex (fire retardant material). If you decide to use the DEET you already have, evidence suggests that 33% is sufficient for protection, and no increase occurs at higher concentrations, though the duration of protection may increase. – US Air Force DEET Fact Sheet.

If You Suspect a reaction to DEET

If you suspect that you or your child is having an adverse reaction to DEET, discontinue use, wash treated skin, and call your local poison control center or physician for help. If you go to a doctor, take the repellent container with you.

More Information

REI Expert Advice on Insect Repellent.

How to Use Insect Repellents Safely

Methods of Mosquito Control

EPA Pesticide Factsheet

National Pesticide Information Center (NPIC) 1-800-858-7378. (Este Web page está disponible en español).

Research

Duke Pharmacologist Says Animal Studies on DEET's Brain Effects Warrant Further Testing and Caution in Human Use

DEET-based insect repellents: safety implications for children and pregnant and lactating women. Koren G, Matsui D, Bailey B.

Neurological effects associated with use of the insect repellent N,N-diethyl-m-toluamide (DEET). Osimitz TG. Murphy JV.

Insect repellant interactions: sunscreens enhance deet (N,N-diethyl-m-toluamide) absorption. Drug Metabolism & Disposition. Ross EA. Savage KA. Utley LJ. Tebbett IR.

Comparative efficacy of insect repellants against mosquito bites. Fradin MS, Day JF.

Evidence for inhibition of cholinesterases in insect and mammalian nervous systems by the insect repellent deet.

18. TRAPS, NETS, COILS & MORE

Here in Thailand my Gecko lizards pounce on any mosquitoes that sneak inside my tightly screened apartment. Even so, I squirt every dark corner and cranny with Baygon, the deadliest insecticide on the planet (and unavailable in the US – probably because its also deadly to humans). If you need more firepower than geckos and insecticide, here are some offensive and defensive weapons:

Mosquito Nets

Product Name & Amazon Link: <u>Moustifluid Impregnated Mousquito Net</u>

- **Sales Pitch:** The Moustifluid Impregnated Mousquito Net for 2 is specially designed fot risky tropical zones. It is suitable for adults, children and pregnant women. It remains effective, against all type of insects, up to 6 months and after 6 washings. Easy to carry thanks to its travel pouch, and easy to use. Composed of only 1 attachment point and a large opening net, it offers a great space and can be set up anywhere for protection against all insects.The net is impregnated the insecticide deltamethrin, recommended by the WHO for protection from infectious diseases carried by insects such as Malaria, Dengue, etc.. The sleeper is protected even in case of direct contact with the net, mosquitoes that may have entered the net when it was opened, and the protection is maintained even if there's a small tear in the net. Floor width: 6 m². Height: 2.50 m. Weight: 450 g. Material: Polyester Tulle Wire: 40 Coins. Mesh: 156 stitches per square inch.

Clothing & Sprays

Name & Link: <u>Zorrel - Insect Shield Apparel Long Sleeve Tee Shirt</u>.

Sales Pitch: Insect Shield® Repellent Apparel and Insect Shield® Repellent Gear are revolutionary products designed to provide long-lasting, effective and convenient personal insect protection. The durable protection provided by Insect Shield apparel and gear is the result of years of research and testing. The U.S. Environmental Protection Agency granted registration of Insect Shield Insect Repellent Apparel--the first-ever, EPA-registered insect-repellent clothing. Recently, EPA has granted Insect Shield extended durability claims for its apparel registration, through 70 washings. Seventy washings is nearly three times the longevity of the original EPA apparel registration at 25 washings. Insect Shield apparel and gear products combine the patent-pending Insect Shield process with a proprietary formulation of the insect repellent permethrin--resulting in effective, odorless insect protection that lasts the expected lifetime of a garment.

Typical Review: By <u>Ella Hill</u> on January 28, 2011

Color Name: HeatherSize Name: Small

This is a unisex shirt (or at least plain enough that we girls can wear it, too, with men's sizing). For reference, I'm tall and usually a women's M and the small fit well -- after the first wash it was a little loose but snug enough for active endeavors. I bought it because the price was lower than other Insect Shield shirts and because I didn't want to be dressed like a 50-year old tourist (camp shirts, awkward fitting button-downs, etc). I just wanted a plain shirt that would work for a variety of outdoor activities. PROS:

- Keeps the bugs away. First tested this out in the rain forest. To be fair, I was also using <u>Insect Repellent</u>. But when I was hiking, everyone who had showered in Deep Woods Off still had a few bites, while I did not. Didn't see any bugs land on me then die, though. It was more like there was a protective bubble around me, while my friends were constantly swatting at bugs.

- Packs well. Bought an extra one that lives rolled up in my bag, just in case (and those cases have been many).

- Dries quickly. Hand washed on a trip and it was dry by morning, even in a humid area. When on, the moisture wicking properties work pretty well, too.

- For the ladies: It doesn't scream "functional clothing." To compare: the Ex Officio Insect Shield shirts look like I went vacation shopping at Orvis. In other words, they might be OK when I'm in the jungle 1000s of miles from home and desperate for a piece of clothing that works, but I wouldn't wear one once I returned home. With the Zorrel one, I can go for a jog, sit out on the patio, etc. (= more uses AND a lower price. Read more ›

Average Score: 4.7/5.0

Name & Link: <u>Sawyer Products Premium Permethrin Clothing Insect Repellent Trigger Spray</u>.

Sales Pitch: As a treatment for clothing, Sawyer Permethrin clothing insect repellent does not harm fabrics and is odorless after dried. Use Permethrin on clothing by itself or with skin-applied repellents to create the ultimate protective, armor-like insect barrier. Permethrin-treatments on clothing are non-toxic to humans and are registered for use by the U.S. EPA. The active ingredient, Permethrin, is a synthetic molecule similar to those found in natural pyrethrum, which is taken from the chrysanthemum flower. Not only does this product repel insects, but will actually kill ticks, mosquitoes, chiggers, mites and more than 55 other kinds of insects. Sawyer Permethrin insect repellents are for use with clothing, tents, and other gear. During the drying process, it tightly bonds with the fibers of the treated garment. It will not stain or damage clothing, fabrics, plastics, finished surfaces, or any of your outdoor gear. Permethrin is a contact insecticide. It kills ticks or other insects when it comes in contact with them. It uses the same active ingredient used in hair shampoos for head lice. When applied to clothing, the Permethrin binds to the fabric eliminating the risk of over-exposure to the skin. As a clothing, tent, chairs, or sleeping bag application, Permethrin is very effective at keeping ticks from attaching to you and at reducing the mosquito population in your camping area. While ticks usually find you at the ankle level (be sure to treat the socks and pants) they can also climb bushes and find you at a higher level so be sure to treat your shirt as well if you are around bushes and concerned about ticks. Permethrin is also an effective repellent against mosquitoes and flies and can be used in conjunction with a skin based repellent.

Typical Review: I pretreated all the clothing I took with me to Haiti with this spray and had no problems with bugs the whole time. I would highly recommend this product to anyone going to areas where malaria would be an issue as well as highly bug inhabited places in the US. I wouldn't use this everyday, but for special occasions - it's a must have. Just make sure you wear gloves when applying and apply exactly as instructed.

Average Score: 4.5/5.0

Mosquito Coils, Incense...

The WHO says mosquito incense should contain d-allethrin in order to be both effective and safe, so read the warnings and instructions before you light up. Mosquito coils have long contained all kinds of cheap toxins added by unregulated manufacturers. US researchers found they often contain heavy metals, allethrin (not the d-form), phenol, and o-cresol – all of which create toxic smoke with adverse effects on humans, which researchers compared the effects to smoking several packs of cigarettes. Doctors caution against the use of mosquito coils for their toxicity and harmful effects on the lungs. On the other hand, I grew up with them. We used them indoors all summer (we had no screens) and all of my family are hale and hearty into their 70s. My mother was still using them at 102. In the Research chapter you'll find an interesting mosquito coil project funded by Bill and Melinda Gates! In the meantime, here's a reputable product that's been well reviewed on Amazon. Click the link for details:

Product Name & Link: Coghlan's 8686 Mosquito Coil.

Sales Pitch: 10 Pack, Mosquito Coil, Kills & Repels Mosquitoes, Each Coil Will Burn 6 Hours Or More, Active Ingredient: 0.23% D-Cis Trans Allethrin, Includes 2 Metal Stands

Typical Review: I had doubted the effectiveness of these mosquito coils for the longest time. I never thought they'd do much for warding off mosquitoes especially outside, where a slight breeze can render most (non-applied) insect repellents useless. These coils, though, work shockingly well...even with a breeze. My wife and I went from literally dozens of bites per evening to barely one or 2. They last quite a long time too. I never timed one, but I can say that they last at least the 6 hours that Coghlan's claims. And if you want to go inside, simply knock off the cherry and you can reuse the remainder of the coil at a later date. They are a must have for anyone with mosquito problems.

Average Score: 4.5/5. **Price**: US$10.00

Standing Water Treatment

Product Name & Link: Mosquito Bits

Sales Pitch: Environmentally sound biological mosquito control; Kills mosquitoes fast, within 24 hours; EPA registered in all 50 states; Sprinkle in any standing water.

Typical Review: I sprinkled some in the pond and started noticing within a few days that mosquitoes couldn't pick up and carry off the dog anymore... after a week, they are almost gone. Sure theres the occasional one or two buzzing around sticking their tongues out at us as they fly by... but I can actually go out and enjoy my garden for a change without taking a bath in DEET first. Very Very VERY pleased with this stuff and I will be buying more every season. Now maybe my neighbors will talk to me and stop contemplating bulldozing my pond over when I'm out of town! Ha!

Average Score: 4.7/5.0. **Price**: $18.00

Product Name & Link: <u>Mosquito Torpedo 300 Day</u>

Sales Pitch: Just Place in Standing Water; Each treatment provides 60 days of protection; No Float design; No unsightly debris; Won't harm humans, animals, fish or vegetation when used as directed

Typical Review: This product is easy to use, effective, and doesn't have particles that float to the surface to mar the beauty of your water feature. I have used the Mosquito Torpedo for several years. **Score:** 4.5/5.0. **Price:** US$14.00

Mosquito Zappers – Stationary

Product Name & Link: <u>Flowtron BK-15D Electronic Insect Killer, 1/2 Acre Coverage</u>

Sales Pitch: Advanced electronic insect control; non clogging killing grid; 1/2-acre killing radius; not to be used within 25-feet of area intended for human activity, should not be attached to house or deck or other structures; instantaneous operation, continuous and uninterrupted service; Uses a 15-watt bulb

- **Typical Review**: These cheap, UV light killers work well indoors if you leave them on overnight in the bedroom. Close doors and windows after dusk because the indoor lights attract mosquitos from miles around after dark.

Score: 4.0/5. **Price**: $28.98

Mosquito Zappers – Handheld for Extra Satisfaction

Product Name, Link: <u>The Executioner PRO Fly Swat Wasp Bug Mosquito Swatter Zapper</u>

- **Sales Pitch:** The Ultimate Fly Zapper , The ExecutionerTM PRO; Bigger, Stronger, Better, Made with ABS Plastic; Supplied Complete with FREE Branded Alkaline Batteries; Fully

CE Approved and Trading Standards Passed, RoHS Compliant; 1 Years Full Warranty, The Best Bug Swatter Available.

Typical Review: The unit activates with a single push button on the handle with a solid click,it must be held in manually. A red led and a high pitched whine let you know it is powered up and ready for business! This thing will kill pretty much whatever it touches in the bug world. It does so with a bright blue flash, and a snap that's louder than several cap guns. By mistake i swung at something at night and it was a bat, and this unit killed it (sorry, it was not intentional, i know bats are useful, my bad). This unit does not have the protective mesh on the racket to protect you from shock, so be careful. This is actually a good thing because it will zap any size creature, whereas the ons that have the protection are limited on the size of the critter they can zap.

Average Score: 4.7/5. **Price**: US$30.00

Home-Made Mosquito Traps

Mosquito Tornado Sucker. Video

Or a simple, passive one like this. (Video)

You'll need

- 1 cup of water
- 1/4 cup of brown sugar
- 1 gram of yeast
- ½ liter bottle

HOW:

1. Cut the plastic bottle in half.

2. Mix brown sugar with hot water. Let cool. When cold, pour in the bottom half of the bottle.

3. Add the yeast. No need to mix. It creates carbon dioxide, which attracts mosquitoes.

4. Place the funnel part, upside down, into the other half of the bottle, taping them together if desired.

5. Wrap the bottle with something black, leaving the top uncovered, and place it outside in an area away from your normal gathering area. (Mosquitoes are also drawn to the color black.)

6. Change the solution every 2 weeks for continuous control.

Professional Mosquito Traps

Product Name & Link: <u>**Flowtron FC-8800 Diplomat Fly Control Device 120Watts Indoor/Outdoor**</u>.

Sales pitch: Control night flying insect up to 2 acres; 120 watts UV lure power covers 1,200 sqft indoors; Mounts vertical or horizontally; For outdoor & commercial indoor us at dumpsters & trash receptacles, barns; Removable collection tray.

- **Typical review:** It's big. It's bad. It's the biggest baddest bug zapping machine you're ever likely to lay hands on, and about as much fun as you can have without committing a felony these days. Seriously, if the machine gun like sound caused by the non stop electrocution of massive quantities of blood sucking pests doesn't cause the joys of boyhood mischief to rise in your heart like a tidal wave of glee, you're already dead. My chickens go ballistic when I bring dead insect catcher to them. A dozen chickens can eat an inch of bugs in the collection pan in about 5 minutes. So I really killed a few birds with one stone on this one. It kills the flys, my wife is getting bit much less and the chickens are getting their fill of insects.

- **Score:** 4.5 stars. **Price:** US$260

Product Name & Link: <u>**Mega-Catch PRO 900 PREMIER XC Mosquito Trap**</u>

Sales Pitch: Programmable timer, infrared energy source, LED display; Can be fine-tuned to target specific mosquito species; Uses less energy than a 40 watt bulb; Self-serviceable with on-board diagnostics.

- **Typical review**: We live in Florida next to a preserve and a lake this is the best thing EVER We even had a follow up call from New Zealand to make sure it was put in the right place. Don't bother with any other companies we really dud our home work and it payed off big time. Just a not you do need to do the three way thing treat the eggs on the grass with insecticide have a repellant near your for the first few week and then it does the rest after 6-8 weeks the breeding cycle is gone A FANTASTIC PRODUCT CAN NOTE RATE HIGHER.
- **Score**: 5/5. **Price:** US$600.

Foggers

Product Name & Link: Burgess 1443 Propane Fogger.

Sales Pitch: Ideal before backyard picnics, barbecques, pool parties and events; Immediate, effective, long lasting control of mosquitoes and flies; Fog in minutes and be bug free for hours; Propane powered for ultimate portability, uses tall canister; 10-foot cone of oderless fog immediately clears bugs from area; 1-year warranty

Typical Review: produces a gloriously sized mosquito-killing cloud of joy. Any slight disappointment about the thickness of the plastic handle is quickly consumed by a thick, lingering, cascading cloud of death and subsequent elation.

- **Score**: 4.7/5.0. **Price:** US$66.

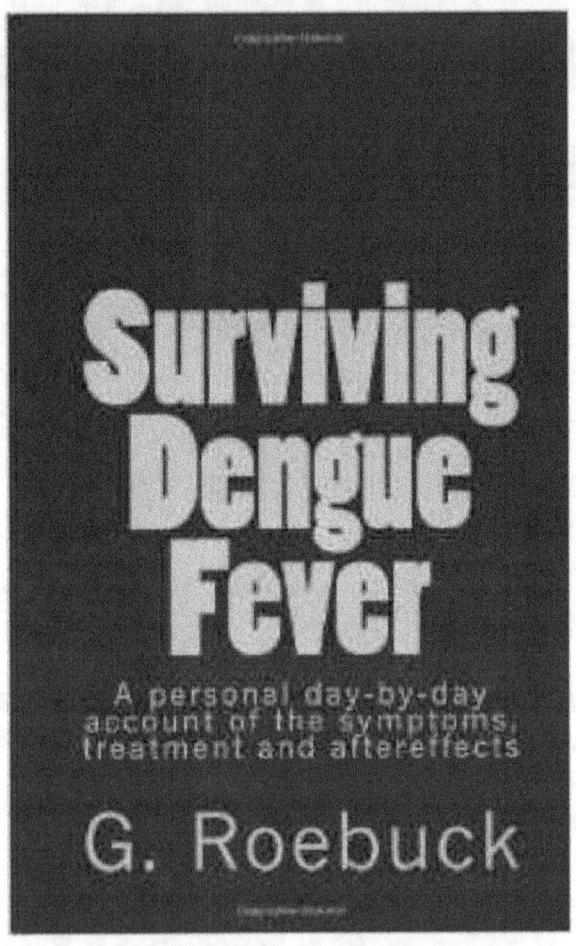

Surviving Dengue Fever: A Personal Day-by-Day Account of the Symptoms, Treatment and Severe Aftereffects by G. Roebuck (**Paperback only**)

Author's Introdution: Surviving Dengue Fever is a factual personal account of what it is like to suffer from this unpleasant tropical disease. Far from being a mild flu-like virus as some sources suggest, this mosquito-borne disease causes unpleasant symptoms and after-effects that linger for months. In more serious cases, Dengue Fever can be fatal.

The author kept a diary of the symptoms, along with the best treatments found to alleviate the fever, rash, painful joints and peeling skin that accompany Dengue fever. Written in simple layman's terms, Surviving Dengue Fever offers an in-depth insight into what to expect if you are unfortunate enough to be contract Dengue fever. It answers many questions that sufferers and their carers may have about Dengue fever, particularly the timeline of each phase of the disease.

It describes the many unexpected after-effects such as peeling skin, hair loss, weight loss and vertigo that the author experienced up to 12 weeks after being diagnosed with Dengue fever. As a handbook, Surviving Dengue Fever gives a full and detailed account of Dengue Fever from the patient's point of view. This invaluable book should be recommended reading for all tropical travelers and medical practitioners who may come into contact with Dengue fever.

- Paperback: 72 pages
- US Price: $6.95
- Publisher: CreateSpace (April 10, 2014)
- Language: English
- ISBN-10: 147524021X
- ISBN-13: 978-1475240214
- Product Dimensions: 8 x 5 x 0.2 inches

Battling Dengue Fever: The Pain and Effort to Cure the Disease

When my husband first showed Dengue symptoms I thought it was 'flu because I had been nursing 'flu since I was in Indonesia. However, as the clock ticked, his high fever rose further. On top of that he had body aches, chills, diarrhea, vomiting, lower stomach pains, zero appetite, rashes all over his body and red eyes. Pain killers from the local doctor didn't help much and the rashes still looked ominous.

On the 3rd day after we returned from Indonesia my husband's condition had not improved so his parents made him go to the hospital. When his blood test revealed that the Dengue virus in his blood was reactive and his blood platelet (thrombocyte) count was below normal (150-450), we had to admit him. Dengue fever can be lethal if not treated fast and properly.

His doctor initially foresaw that my husband would need to stay in the hospital 3-4 days to cure his Dengue. However, after 4 days in the hospital my husband's condition worsened so his stay had to be extended. Spending 6-11 hours a day in the hospital to look after him was my new routine. I was pregnant at the time and not supposed to get too tired but it's just not easy to leave your husband alone in the hospital!

Every day during his hospitalization my parents, his parents and I hoped and tried to raise his platelet count. Because we were aware that Dengue virus would make his platelet count drop we attempted to manage the fall to be above 50, otherwise he would need to be put in the ICU or given blood transfusions. And while his doctor had given him IV drips to give him enough fluid, we had to force him to drink plenty of liquids to keep his blood cells intact.

One time my husband's condition turned pretty bad: his platelet count plunged to its lowest level, 57! and he had a sudden onset of high fever. By then, asking my husband to drink plain water or other drinks was like nailing jelly to a wall. Furthermore, his doctor said there is no exact cure for Dengue fever but pain killers, total bed rest and lots of water. His body has to fight the Dengue virus by itself. When my parents in Indonesia figured that my husband's condition had worsened, they thought of taking the first flight to Malaysia on the next day to see him but I managed to assure them that I still could handle it alone.

Believe it or not, my Mother-in-Law and I tried to find, make and give my husband all of the following natural remedies and alternative Chinese medicines, hoping to arrest his plummeting platelet count. We learned the information below from my parents, relatives, friends and even the hospital's nurse as they had successfully treated Dengue fever with one or few of these alternative solutions on top of doctor's clinical treatment:

1. **Pink Guava Juice** – This juice is believed to have properties in cell repair and to be high in iron and vitamin C. It's traditionally used for treating Dengue fever in Indonesia. I personally think the juice tastes nice but my husband hated it.

2. **Red Dates (hong zhao) and Red Yeast Rice (angkak) Tea** – Our family doctor in Indonesia himself suggested that he consume plenty of this tea because it can increase platelets. My husband drank red dates and honey tea for two days before he refused to drink it any more.

3. **Coconut Water** – This drink is cooling and replenishes electrolytes, minerals plus other

trace minerals lost by the body due to dehydration.

4. **Isotonic Drink** – My husband's doctor and nurses themselves advised my husband repeatedly to take an isotonic drink to keep his body hydrated but he always declined and asked me to throw away the isotonic drinks I bought for him.

5. **Papaya Leaves' Juice** – It is believed that papaya leaves contain substances responsible for the production of platelets. Papaya leaves' extract is usually used to treat severe Dengue fever and possesses incredibly bitter taste. My husband took few sips of this and his platelet counts increased a little bit on the following day.

6. **Bitter gourd and Frog Leg Soup** – I am not so sure of the health benefits of this soup but it's well known in the Chinese community in Malaysia for controlling Dengue fever. It's bitter and not easy to drink. My husband vomited twice after consuming it.

7. **Crab Soup (Sup Ketam)** – One of the hospital nurses suggested we make this for my husband as it's rich in protein and commonly used by the Malay community to overcome Dengue. My Mom-in-Law boiled this soup for my husband but he did not even bother to taste it because it's obviously one smelly soup!

8. **Palm Dates (Kurma)** – Dates are high in sugar, zinc, vitamins and cure intestinal disturbances. My Dad suggested introducing this to my husband especially since my husband once complained that he had gastric pain due to his poor eating patterns in the hospital. My husband ate dates like a snack and I am not sure if eating these actually contributed to his recovery from Dengue but my husband got better after eating few dates. In my opinion, food that has been consumed for thousand years, potentially since the Biblical era, like dates - are not eaten for nothing. There must be tons of health benefits from them. Thus, I made my husband eat dates as much as he could.

9. **Fu Fang Compound E-Jiao Jiang** – This is a traditional Chinese medicine used for nourishing blood. Based on my Indonesian friends' and relatives' testimonies, their platelet

counts almost immediately increased after drinking this medicine - so we tried it on my husband too. It's easy to purchase in most Chinese herbs shops in Indonesia but not so easy to find in Malaysia.

It was hard to make him drink lots of water or eat his food but, as his condition improved, he drank more water on his own and could request specific foods when he felt hungry.

On the sixth day in the hospital his platelet count was already above 100 but his doctor did not want to release him just yet as my husband's body, especially his hands, were so swollen and reddish. Seemingly, my husband had experienced bleeding underneath his skin which normally only occurs to people with platelet counts below 50. Therefore, his doctor said that he needed to carefully observe him longer to make sure he didn't bleed from his lungs, mouth, nose, etc..

At last, after total of 7 days of hospitalization, his platelet count was back in normal range and his fever, chills and body pains lessened. The swelling and redness on his hands had somewhat reduced (but not completly gone) and his doctor gave him the green light to rest at home with a note that he has to take medical leave for at least one more week.

So I am delighted to announce that my sleepless nights and running in and out plus standing by in the hospital for hours came to an end. I've got my husband back at home with me now, even though he is still not fully recovered. He is still red, weak and clearly, much thinner. Seeing your partner sick and in so much pain was indeed painful but I am glad that everything turned better.

To finish this post I'll pass on this advice from an officer of the local Ministry of Health (MoH) who visited us in the hospital: do remember to remove stagnant clean water in your premises at all times and use mosquitoes spray in your house twice a day to prevent the *Aedes Aegypti* mosquitos from breeding. Don't get bitten! By the way, a day after this government officer's visit in the hospital, there was a team sent by MoH spraying mosquito's pesticides around our Seremban house's residential area. Isn't that good! – Follow Christine's adventures at her blog, The Wanderer's Journal.

20. TRANSMISSION

To spark a more severe Dengue outbreak you need three things. First, imported virus: check. Second, a population with no immunity. The United States has that, since Dengue was last widespread in the 1940s. Third, mosquitoes that can transmit it. Those are already widespread. – Science writer Maryn Mckenna.

Dengue is surprisingly vulnerable to human intervention in its life cycle. Break any link in the chain and Dengue transmission stops. Here are some potential intervention stages:

1. Uninfected female *Aedes* finds feverish Dengue-infected human.

2. *Aedes* bites feverish Dengue human.

3. *Aedes* hides and rests for 3-4 days.

4. Dengue virus moves into the *Aedes'* salivary glands.

5. *Aedes* lays eggs in water.

6. Dengue-infected *Aedes* finds and bites human.

7. Mosquito eggs hatch, develop into adults in 4-7 days in tropics.

8. Newly hatched female mosquito has sex with male mosquitoes.

9. Infected female looks for new blood meals, infecting those she bites.

Break One Link
in the Dengue Transmission Chain
and Transmission Ends

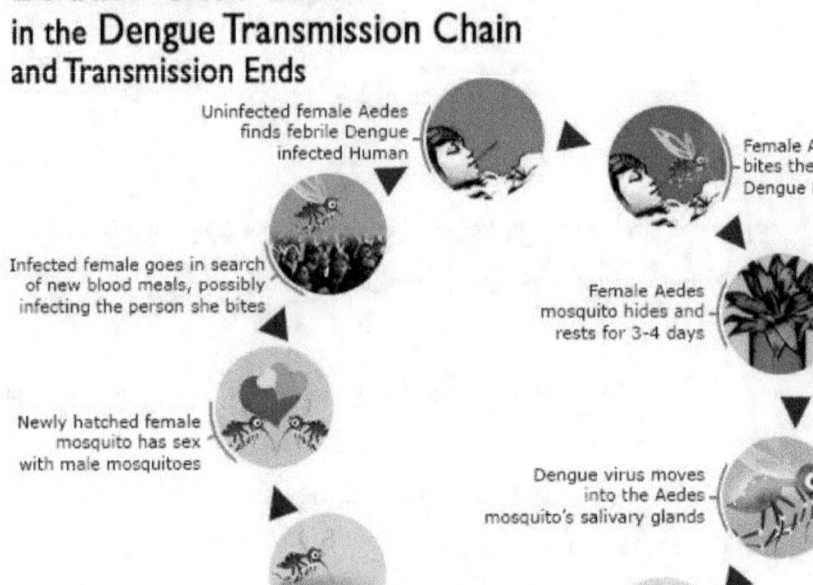

Uninfected female Aedes finds febrile Dengue infected Human

Female Aedes bites the febrile Dengue Human

Infected female goes in search of new blood meals, possibly infecting the person she bites

Female Aedes mosquito hides and rests for 3-4 days

Newly hatched female mosquito has sex with male mosquitoes

Dengue virus moves into the Aedes mosquito's salivary glands

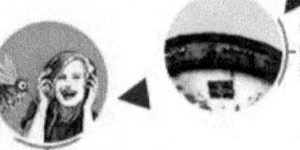

Mosquito eggs hatch and develop into adults in 7 days in tropical temperatures

Female Aedes mosquito lays eggs in water

The now Dengue-infected female Aedes mosquito finds human and bites human

Credit
World Health
Organization

21. VACCINES, BACTERIA & GMOS

Research from scientists at the University of Queensland in Australia has found that when *Aedes*
Aegypti mosquitoes are infected with a bacteria called Wolbachia they can only make babies after
drinking human blood. Guinea pigs, mice, sheep, pigs and chickens just aren't good enough.
Biological controls are wonderful when they work but expensive to develop because biological
systems are so variable and adaptive. So it's no surprise that humans have collectively spent almost
$1 billion on Dengue vectors with, thus far, zero success.

Vaccines

The good news is that, since Dengue has spread to rich countries, researchers have been able to
raise enough money to test non-toxic ways of preventing the disease. The IFPMA (International
Federation of Pharmaceutical Manufacturers & Associations), in the search for vaccines against so-
called Neglected Tropical Diseases, using 2010 as the baseline aim, by 2020, to reduce Dengue
mortality and morbidity by 50% and 25% respectively.

The prevalence of the strains varies geographically, but all four are commonly found in endemic
areas. The scientific challenge is to develop a vaccine that elicits an immune response against all
four serotypes.

Sanofi-Pasteur is the vaccine division of $40 billion Sanofi Pharmaceuticals. They've spent 10 years
and $500 million developing a Dengue fever vaccine. They've been carrying out Phase 3 trials with
31,000 children and adolescents in Mexico, Colombia, Honduras, Puerto Rico, Brazil, the
Philippines, Vietnam, Malaysia, Indonesia, and Thailand.

- They're so confident of success that they've already built a new plant to manufacture the vaccine in Neuville-sur-Saône, France. They think they have a blockbuster on their hands because

- It seems to work on 3 serotypes, DV1, DV3, & DV4, cutting infection rates by 55% for serotype 1, 75% for serotype 3, and 100% for serotype 4
- No previous attempts at Dengue vaccines have worked against even one strain.
- It seems to be safe.
- Though it might cause some common vaccination responses, it doesn't cause serious Dengue.

Before we get our hopes up, let's see why some experts urge caution:

- It requires 3 injections.
- It will cost $10–$50 per shot, a fortune in most tropical countries.
- It is only effective for 30 days. We need lifetime protection.
- It didn't work on Thailand's most common strain, Serotype 2, when tested on 4,000 Thai children.

Bacteria (the Good Kind)

For reasons we don't understand, mosquitoes that feed on human blood have better health and produce more offspring than mosquitoes fed on other kinds of animal blood. So how could simple bacteria break this cycle?

The *Wolbachia* bacterium is found in many insects, including fruit flies but, for reasons not fully understood, is not naturally carried by *Aedes*.

Australian scientist Scott O'Neill has been working with *Wolbachia* for 20 years and, in 2008, had a breakthrough. One of his research students implanted the bacteria in a mosquito so that it could be passed on to future generations. As they watched, they saw that the *Wolbachia*-infected mosquitoes died quicker *and* – partially or completely – blocked Dengue infection in the mosquito, like a natural vaccine.

O'Neill, now dean of science at Monash University, Melbourne, says, "If Dengue can't grow in the mosquito, it can't be transmitted." In lab trials Dengue was found in only 4.2% of saliva samples taken from the *Wolbachia*-infected mosquitoes compared to 80.2% of saliva samples taken from "unprotected" mosquitoes.

There are now large scale field trials in Brazil using *Wolbachia* bacteria to infect female *Aedes*. But, as with the vaccine, there are some big hurdles to be overcome before we can hope to benefit from it:

- It is not clear exactly how *Wolbachia* guards mosquitoes from Dengue infection, but studies indicate that *Wolbachia* infection seemingly boosts or manipulates the mosquito's immune system to interfere with replication of the Dengue virus.

- Trials suggest that *Wolbachia* infection must reach a critical, minimum level in order to guard against Dengue infection.

- It's possible that over time, as a mosquito species becomes adapted to Wolbachia infection, the corresponding protection against Dengue may wear off. It seems that this may have happened with a close cousin, *Aedes albopictus.*

- *Wolbachia* currently provides protection against only serotype 2. Can it protect against the other 3 Dengue serotypes?

The bad news:

- A pilot program to eliminate Dengue fever on a small island in central Vietnam failed after initial success, according to results presented at an international conference on Wednesday.

- A population of Dengue fever-carrying mosquitoes implanted with Wolbachia (a bacteria known to suppress the virus) has almost disappeared, Tuoi Tre (Youth) newspaper reported. Around 800 families living on the south-central Khanh Hoa Province's Dengue fever hot spot received Aedes aegypti larvae infected with the bacteria in April of last year.

- The project team hoped that the Wolbachia-carrying mosquitoes would become the dominant aedes aegypti community on the island in three months and go on to eliminate the disease in the area and the country.
- But six months after their release, their population began to plummet.
- "Early results indicated success, but after a while, the [modified] mosquito community almost disappeared," Vice Minister of Health Nguyen Thanh Long announced at the conference held in Nha Trang, the capital resort town of Khanh Hoa.
- **Members of the project team told conference attendees that only one percent of the 8,000 larvae they introduced on Tri Nguyen island have survived.** Dengue mitigation pilot fails on Vietnam island.

But I kept seeing positive reports about Wolbachia trials so, once again, I asked Steve Fry, a scientist himself, living in a heavily-infected Dengue area, and whose partner is a world authority on Dengue. (What better combination could you ask for?). Here's the correspondence:

To: Steve,

Do you have any idea whether this approach has been fruitful in earlier trials? I get mixed reports.
– Godfree

Hi Godfree,

The results for Wolbachia infected mosquito release programs have been a mixed bag. They sort-worked in the first Australian field trials - but not as well as hoped-for. The second big round of tests/usage/programs in Vietnam - with lots of early and on-going positive press coverage and positive press releases - but the realities have been that the releases of Wolbachia infected mosquitoes have NOT ultimately created large enough populations to affect Dengue infection rates in meaningful ways - and the releases of Wolbachia infected mosquitoes have also not even produced self-sustaining populations. Still, the scientists and govts who advocate using them are hopeful, while the data and results say this idea is "no where near ready for prime time". The Wolbachia infected mosquito release programs will ultimately remain failures, as long as:

1. The proportions of wolbachia infected mosquitoes remain too small to be effective, and

2. The populations of wolbachia infectted mosquitoes remain non-sustaining.

It's possible that the problems can be resolved, but there has not been much significant progress (approaching success) in the past 8 years. I am not against the approach, but just note that   we need programs that work.   http://www.scidev.net/asia-pacific/health/news/setback-for-dengue-blocking-mosquito-trial-in-vietnam.html

Note that programs for eliminating mosquito breeding grounds have worked for eliminating mosquito vectors of human disease - like the elimination of Yellow Fever for example - but it takes the resolve and efforts of both govt. and people.

Over 110 years of clever science and cute science and scientific claims are all very seductive - and very promising - but so far they have not worked in this area- ... while good old-fashioned   elbow-grease efforts are proven to work across many cultures and many nations....   But... it takes resolve, persistence, and consensus - and historically it also takes government enforcement.

In contrast to the Yellow Fever success,   instead consider how Dengue was completely eradicated from the Americas (the whoe western Hemisphere) except for the laziness and lying of Cuban leaders....   Castro and his jerks lied and lied and lied about their mosquito control efforts for over a decade - and those jerks imprisoned and ruined any Cuban scientist or physician who publicly disagreed with them...   And that Cuban Dengue reservoir has needlessly gone on to infect the Americas, again.

GMOs: Sterile Insects

Four different serotypes represent a challenge to vaccines, which is why genetic modification looks promising: it simply eradicates *Aedes* regardless of the serotype.

The Sterile Insect Technique (SIT) is well known, well understood and, when it works, works well. It eradicated screw-worm, a cattle pest, in North America and has reduced populations of pests like Tsetse fly in Zanzibar. SIT uses the natural instincts of released, sterile male mosquitoes to seek out females, so it is much more effective than traditional means at targeting difficult-to-reach pests like *Aedes*, which hides in homes. It's also species-specific: it affects only the target pest and doesn't harm other insects or humans.

But the traditional approach of using radiation to produce sterile insects isn't very good for them! Often, irradiated males are sickly (who wouldn't be after microwaving?), so wild females reject them. Mosquitoes are delicate and easily damaged by irradiation, so to date there have been no successful programs of mosquito control using radiation-based SIT.

British biotech firm, Oxitec, have developed a strain of *Aedes,* poetically named OX513A, to carry a gene that produces a protein which, when passed on, kills the next generation of mosquitoes while they're still larvae. With typical British cunning they've engineered the gene so that the drug tetracycline prevents production of the deadly protein.

They raise healthy mosquitoes in the lab by adding a pinch of tetracycline to the larvae's diet. Then, in the wild, without tetracycline, mosquito offspring inheriting the gene die as larvae.

The idea is to flood the air with genetically-modified males that will mate with females in the wild. The resulting offspring that inherit the lethal gene from their GM fathers will die – leading to a population crash. Oxitec calls this strategy Release of Insects carrying a Dominant Lethal (RIDL). You could think of the males as being effectively sterile.

In 2010, field tests of RIDL conducted in the Cayman Islands demonstrated that the strategy was effective in <u>driving down the island population of A. aegypti by 80%</u>. Trials in Brazil achieved 96% suppression in 2013. Here's Oxitec's press report from Brazil:

Moscamed (the mosquito control authority) announced that they had achieved a 96% reduction of the adult mosquito population in the target area the village of Mandacarú, in north-eastern Brazil. Over the course of 6 months, Moscamed periodically released male OX513A mosquitoes into the target area. The males (which don't bite) mated with wild females, passing on a lethal gene to their offspring and, in effect, preventing them from having viable offspring. The effect on the local population of the Dengue vector was dramatic: analysis of eggs laid in specially designed 'ovitraps' showed that the number of viable 'wild-type' eggs laid in the trial areas was reduced by 91-95%, while adult trapping showed a reduction in the local adult population of an estimated 96%. The isolated location of the target area enabled an even greater level of suppression than achieved previously, something that Oxitec's Dr Luke Alphey finds very encouraging: "In this trial we've seen that when releases are carried out in a relatively isolated area, our approach leads to even greater population reduction than we have reported previously, as immigration from neighboring areas is reduced. This also indicates that in the right conditions, local elimination of a target pest species should be possible."

Mosquito control officials in Florida have requested FDA approval to use genetically-modified mosquitoes to eradicate *Aedes* populations in the Florida Keys. So this approach seems to be gaining ground.

The sober truth is that, though all of these approaches may work for a while, only when we combine efforts to stop *Aedes* breeding can offer permanent Dengue reductions, as we learned in Cuba and other places. No mosquitoes = no Dengue.

22. REGULAR MOSQUITO BITES

Most mosquito bites don't result in Dengue but they're a nuisance, uncomfortable for people with allergic reactions and, when children scratch them, can lead to infections. Here are some strategies if you want to stop the itching and scratching:

- Cooling with ice helps for a short time.
- Put hot water – as hot as you can bear it – on the affected area.
- Train a hair dryer on the new bite as hot as you can tolerate for as long as you can bear it. The high temperature destroys most of the itch enzymes. I bought a cheap little hair dryer just for mosquito bite itch. It works fine.
- To take the sting out, either apply a poultice of equal parts brown sugar and liquid dish washing soap or rub the bite with a moist bar of soap. For major itching, dab on some menthol or spearmint toothpaste.
- Ask your pharmacist for a cream containing Chlorphenoxamine, an antihistamine, and apply a small amount. It removes the itching and swelling within minutes.
- Ask the pharmacist for a cream containing Betamethasone, a powerful glucocorticoid steroid with anti-inflammatory and immunosuppressive properties.

23. YOUR COMMUNITY

Since 2001, three autochthonous [indigenous] dengue fever outbreaks have occurred in the United States: in Hawaii (2001); Brownsville, Texas (2005); and southern Florida (2009–2011).

After analyzing the 3 outbreaks, we found the following prominent themes in the response efforts:

1. timely detection of illness;

2. communication of up-to-date, correct information; and

3. development of a rapid response that engages the community.

We therefore recommend that public health authorities involve the clinical and laboratory community promptly, provide accurate information, and engage the local community in vector control and case identification and reporting. – CDC

If you're moved to action in your community, here's the most recent information:

WHO's 5-Step Community Dengue Program.

The World Health Organization is responsible for the health of everyone on earth. They see more Dengue reports than anyone. Here are their recommendation for communities that want to eradicate Dengue:

1. Advocate, mobilize and legislate to ensure that public health bodies and communities are strengthened;

2. Collaborate between your health department and other public and private sectors;

3. Integrate your approach to disease control to maximize use of resources;

4. Make decisions based on evidence to ensure your interventions are targeted appropriately. For example, generalized spraying with organophosphate or pyrethroid insecticides, while sometimes done, is not thought to be effective, even though it's widely practiced.

5. Build your community's capacity to respond to your local situation.

How the World Bank Sees Dengue

Just 10 years ago in Latin America Dengue was on its way out: only 267,000 cases and just 70 deaths were reported. But between January and May 2009, Argentina suffered the worst outbreak of Dengue in its history.

- The virus quickly spread through 16 provinces. Over 26,000 people fell ill and five died. "A Dengue case every 15 minutes" was the statistic that made the news headlines. However, the following year's numbers reflected a completely different reality: just 900 cases of Dengue were reported in 2010, and since then, not a single death has been attributed to the disease. But Dengue did not just magically disappear.

- The Ministry of Health's national and provincial offices implemented a comprehensive strategy with support from the World Bank and PAHO [Pan-American Health ORganization]/W.H.O.

- A massive epidemiological surveillance system was established: the immediate reporting of cases, timely treatment (in several areas around the country), installation of emergency care tents, the necessary investment in logistics and supplies to eliminate mosquito breeding grounds, as well as a large-scale public awareness campaign to stem the epidemic.

- Carlos Cairo, a coordinator at the Argentine Ministry of Health, said that, "in the fight against Dengue, the key is cultural change, both in the health teams and the communities." Thus, people agreed to the *descacharizado* effort – to eliminate containers that could store water where the mosquito deposits its larvae. Additionally, health care professionals were empowered to diagnose and provide treatment quickly.

- "The way to ensure fewer cases is to make a pact with society," added the World Bank's Fernando Lavadenz, who says that the economic costs of Dengue go well beyond health system costs. Although Dengue no longer makes headlines in Argentina, it is still causing headaches in neighboring countries: last year, Paraguay recorded more than 150,000 cases and 233 deaths whereas Brazil had 1.5 million cases and 456 deaths. Read More...

Dengue and The Red Cross

Dengue is preventable and evidence shows it can be contained. During the 1950s and 1960s a strategy adopted by the Pan-American Health Organization to remove *Aedes aegypti,* the vector responsible for Dengue transmission, successfully reduced and in certain cases eliminated Dengue in the Americas. We need a renewed commitment to integrated programming that includes

1. improved management and diagnosis,
2. increased awareness and community participation in controlling the vector and
3. enhanced environmental sanitation.
4. We aim to prevent Dengue from ever returning to today's level. – Dengue: Turning up the Volume on a Silent Disaster. 23 pages. Downloadable free at www.dengue.us.

A Case Study of Dengue Mosquito Control

VECTOR CONTROL: Surveillance, prevention and control of Dengue in Madeira. A case study of community and public health after a disastrous outbreak of Dengue in Spain.

24. BLOGS, LINKS, DOWNLOADS

Dr. Steven M. Fry, who goes by 'Steve' on his blog, represents a remarkable level of access to, and understanding of, Dengue-related matters. He's a scientist and, as he says, an Environmental and Public Health chemist who's been performing both academic and private laboratory investigations of pesticides, industrial and radiological contaminants and their Public Health consequences since 1976. Even better, he's married to a scientist who studies Dengue full-time. So if you hear a Dengue-related rumor or have a Dengue-related question, head straight to Steve's blog, YucaLandia/Surviving Yucatan.

Beyond Pesticides. A wonderful, tightly focused website created by heavyweight practitioners and scientists like Warren Porter, Ph.D., Professor of Zoology and Environmental Toxicology at the University of Wisconsin at Madison. Dr. Porter's recent research links pesticide exposure in utero to impaired learning, changes in brain function and altered thyroid levels. His lab has also shown lawn chemical mixtures at low-levels increase abortion rates in lab animals.

And, of course, visit Dengue.us and share your misery (and your case history, *please*) with fellow-sufferers!

Also, be sure to download **Dengue - Guidelines for Diagnosis, Treatment, Prevention and Control**. (October 2009), 160 pages. W.H.O.

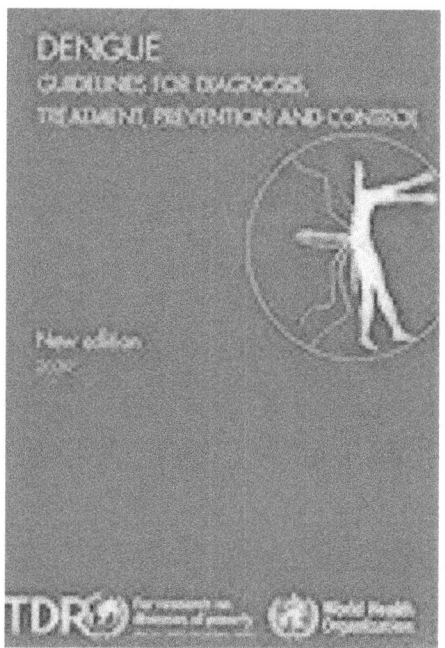

Download the full report here.

25. MYTHS & RUMORS

1. **There's a vaccine for Dengue.** Not yet. Sanofi is working on one (see the *Vaccine* chapter) but it won't be ready to market for some years.

2. **Dengue mosquitos breed in sewers and rivers. It's a'dirty' disease.** Not at all. *Aedes aegepti* breeds happily in old tires and bottle caps in your back yard.

3. **Dengue mosquitos attack at night.** Nope. Though *Aedes* can bite any time, it's most active around dawn and dusk and will happily bite you inside the house or out.

4. **Dengue causes depression.** Like any bout of severe illness, a Dengue infection predisposes you to depression but it doesn't 'cause' depression.

5. **Dengue is a rural disease.** It's much more common in urban and suburban areas.

6. **All mosquitos can carry Dengue**. No. *Aedes* is the carrier of 99% of Dengue infections. But it's wise to behave as if this myth were true because you probably won't know which mosquito bit you until it's too late!

7. **Drinking lots of water prevents DHF/DSS symptoms**. Some doctors still believe this but there's no clinical evidence and no sound scientific reason why it should.

8. **It takes 10+ days between being bitten and the onset of fever & symptoms**. Recent reports indicate an incubation period as short as 4 days between the mosquito bite and the Dengue infection. Read more...

Bogus Cures

A team of Queensland scientists led by microbiologist professor Max Reynolds have developed the world's first cure for Dengue fever by distilling Melaleuca alternifolia leaves from Australia's native tea tree plant. Now available worldwide, 98alive is a unique natural medicine containing Melaleuca alternifolia leaf concentrate that's antiviral, antibacterial and immune boosting properties have been scientifically proven to cure all four strains of Dengue fever.

Anyone claiming to cure Dengue is, at present, a fraud. 98alive is no exception. Even the Queensland, Australia, Health Department has raised a red flag about 98alive.

Right now, we're stuck with treating the symptoms until there's a tested, final solution to the Dengue problem.

26. VIDEOS

If you're lying in bed – or just plain curious about Dengue – here are some YouTube videos to fill the gaps in your Dengue knowledge. Some have excellent animation:

The Dengue Channel: Dengue case studies.

Dengue: turning up the volume on a silent disaster. Dramatic animated graphics about Dengue statistics world wide. Red Cross.

Mosquito Week, with Bill Gates: Bill Gates talks about why he's donated millions to mosquito control.

The Dengue Virus Close Up: Microbiologist Shannon Bennett up close and personal with the virus.

Dengue Virus Infection: Closeup look at the mosquito and the virus.

Aedes: the Dengue Mosquito in Action: Aedes feeding.

Singapore: All about Dengue: great microphotography of the mosquito life cycle.

Dengue prevention in Singapore: Singapore's campaign to fight Dengue fever from spreading in the city.

Severe Dengue (Hemorragic) Fever Treatment: Diagnosing and treating severe Dengue.

Preparing papaya leaf: How to make a batch of papaya leaf juice.

Papaya leaf case study: No sound track

Make a mosquito fan trap: Do it yourself

Dengue: The next vaccine preventable disease?. Sanofi-Pasteur's vaccine in development.

27. DENGUE FOR MDS

If you're a physician and unfamiliar with Dengue, a quick scan of these pages and downloads will bring up up to speed.

Case Management

The Centers for Disease Control has a quick-reference chart for **Dengue case menagement that you can download here**.

Clinical Guidance

The CDC has also produced a complete clinical guide, which you can read here, on their site. I've also reproduced it, below, in case you're away from your computer:

Dengue Virus: Dengue infection is caused by any one of four distinct but closely related Dengue virus (DENV) serotypes (called DENV-1, -2, -3, and -4). These Dengue viruses are single-stranded RNA viruses that belong to the family Flaviviridae and the genus Flavivirus--a family which includes other medically important vector-borne viruses (e.g., West Nile virus, Yellow Fever virus, Japanese Encephalitis virus, St. Louis Encephalitis virus, etc.). Dengue viruses are arboviruses (arthropod-borne virus) that are transmitted primarily to humans through the bite of an infected Aedes species mosquito. Transmission may also occur through transfusion of infected blood or transplantation of infected organs or tissues. Human transmission of Dengue is also known to occur after occupational exposure in healthcare settings (e.g., needle stick injuries) and cases of vertical transmission have been described in the literature (i.e., transmission from a Dengue infected pregnant mother to her fetus in utero or to her infant during labor and delivery).

Clinical Dengue: Infection with any of the four Dengue serotypes can produce the full spectrum of illness and severity. The spectrum of illness can range from a mild, non-specific febrile syndrome to classic Dengue fever (DF), to the severe forms of the disease, Dengue hemorrhagic fever (DHF) and Dengue shock syndrome (DSS). Severe forms typically manifest after a two to seven day febrile phase and are often heralded by clinical and laboratory warning signs. Early clinical recognition of Dengue infection and anticipatory treatment for those who develop DHF or DSS can save lives. While no therapeutic agents exist for Dengue infections, the key to the successful management is timely and judicious use of supportive care, including administration of isotonic intravenous fluids or colloids, and close monitoring of vital signs and hemodynamic status, fluid balance, and hematologic parameters. (Recommended therapies and treatment courses for DF, DHF and DSS can be found at the links provided below.)

As the early presentations of DF and DHF/DSS are similar and the course of infection is short, timely identification of persons that will develop severe manifestations can be challenging. There is a long-standing debate as to whether DHF/DSS represents a separate pathophysiological process or is merely the opposite end of a continuum of the same illness. DF follows an uncomfortable but relatively benign self-limited course. DHF may appear as a relatively benign infection at first but can quickly develop into life-threatening illness as fever abates. DHF can usually be distinguished from DF as it progresses through its three predictable pathophysiological phases:

- Febrile phase: Viremia-driven high fevers
- Critical/plasma leak phase: Sudden onset of varying degrees of plasma leak into the pleural and abdominal cavities
- Convalescence or reabsorption phase: Sudden arrest of plasma leak with concomitant reabsorption of extravasated plasma and fluids.

For optimal management of the patient with Dengue infection, it is important to understand these phases and to be able to distinguish DHF from DF. Early recognition of a patient's clinical phase is important in order to tailor clinical management, monitor effectiveness of the treatment, and to anticipate when changes in their management are needed.

Dengue infected patients are either asymptomatic or they have one of three clinical presentations:

- Undifferentiated Fever;
- Dengue Fever with or without hemorrhage; or
- Dengue Hemorrhagic Fever or Dengue Shock Syndrome.

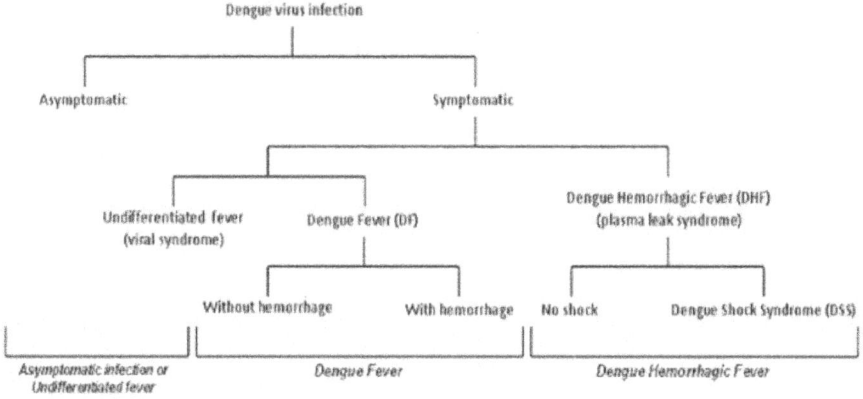

*Adapted from Dengue Haemorrhagic Fever: Diagnosis, Treatment, Prevention and Control. 2nd edition. WHO, Geneva, 1997

Asymptomatic Infection: As many as one half of all Dengue infected individuals are asymptomatic, that is, they have no clinical signs or symptoms of disease.

Undifferentiated Fever: The first clinical course is a relatively benign scenario where the patient experiences fever with mild non-specific symptoms that can mimic any number of other acute febrile illnesses. They do not meet case definition criteria for DF. The non-specific presentation of symptoms make positive diagnosis difficult based on physical exam and routine tests alone. For the majority of these patients, unless Dengue diagnostic serological or molecular testing is performed, the diagnosis will remain unknown. These patients are typically young children or those experiencing their first infection, and they recover fully without need for hospital care.

Dengue Fever with or without hemorrhage: The second clinical presentation occurs when a patient develops DF with or without hemorrhage. These patients are typically older children or adults and they present with two to seven days of high fever (occasionally biphasic) and two or more of the following symptoms: severe headache, retro-orbital eye pain, myalgias, arthralgias, a diffuse erythematous maculo-papular rash, and mild hemorrhagic manifestation. Subtle, minor epithelial hemorrhage, in the form of petechiae, are often found on the lower extremities (but may occur on buccal mucosa, hard and soft palates and or subconjunctivae as well), easy bruising on the skin, or the patient may have a positive tourniquet test. Other forms of hemorrhage such as epistaxis, gingival bleeding, gastrointestinal bleeding, or urogenital bleeding can also occur, but are rare. Leukopenia is frequently found and may be accompanied by varying degrees of thrombocytopenia.

Children may also present with nausea and vomiting. Patients with DF do not develop substantial plasma leak (hallmark of DHF and DSS, see below) or extensive clinical hemorrhage. Serological testing for anti-Dengue IgM antibodies or molecular testing for Dengue viral RNA or viral isolation can confirm the diagnosis, but these tests often provide only retrospective confirmation, as results are typically not available until well after the patient has recovered.

Clinical presentation of DF and the early phase of DHF are similar, and therefore it can be difficult to differentiate between the two forms early in the course of illness. With close monitoring of key indicators, the development of DHF can be detected at the time of defervescence so that early and appropriate therapy can be initiated. The key to successfully managing patients with Dengue infection and lowering the probability of medical complications or death due to DHF or DSS is early recognition and anticipatory treatment. (For more detailed guidance on management for DF please see the recommended treatment courses for DHF in the links listed below.)

Dengue Hemorrhagic Fever (DHF) or Dengue Shock Syndrome (DSS): The third clinical presentation results in the development of DHF, which in some patients progresses to DSS. Vigilant is critical for identifying warning signs of progressing illness and early symptoms of DHF which are very similar to those of DF. Case Definitions Page

There are three phases of DHF:

1. Febrile Phase
2. Critical (Plasma Leak) Phase
3. Convalescent (Reabsorption) Phase.

Febrile Phase: Early in the course of illness, patients with DHF can present much like DF, but they may also have hepatomegaly without jaundice (later in the Febrile Phase). The hemorrhagic manifestations that occur in the early course of DHF most frequently consist of mild hemorrhagic manifestations as in DF. Less commonly, epistaxis, bleeding of the gums, or frank gastrointestinal bleeding occur while the patient is still febrile (gastrointestinal bleeding may commence at this point, but commonly does not become apparent until a melenic stool is passed much later in the course). Dengue viremia is typically highest in the first three to four days after onset of fever but then falls quickly to undetectable levels over the next few days. The level of viremia and fever usually follow each other closely, and anti-Dengue IgM anti-bodies increase as fever abates.

Critical (Plasma Leak) Phase: About the time when the fever abates, the patient enters a period of highest risk for developing the severe manifestations of plasma leak and hemorrhage. At this time, it is vital to watch for evidence of hemorrhage and plasma leak into the pleural and abdominal cavities and to implement appropriate therapies replacing intravascular losses and stabilizing effective volume. If left untreated, this can lead to intravascular volume depletion and cardiovascular compromise. Evidence of plasma leak includes sudden increase in hematocrit ($\geq$20% increase from baseline), presence of ascites, a new pleural effusion on lateral decubitus chest x-ray, or low serum albumin or protein for age and sex. Patients with plasma leak should be monitored for early changes in hemodynamic parameters consistent with compensated shock such as increased heart rate (tachycardia) for age especially in the absence of fever, weak and thready pulse, cool extremities, narrowing pulse pressure (systolic blood pressure minus diastolic blood pressure <20 mmHg), delayed capillary refill (>2 seconds), and decrease in urination (i.e., oliguria). Patients exhibiting signs of increasing intravascular depletion, impending or frank shock, or severe hemorrhage should be admitted to an appropriate level intensive care unit for monitoring and intravascular volume replacement. Once a patient experiences frank shock he or she will be categorized as having DSS. Prolonged shock is the main factor associated with complications that can lead to death including massive gastrointestinal hemorrhage. Interestingly, many patients with DHF/DSS remain alert and lucid throughout the course of the illness, even at the tipping point of profound shock. See case definition for DHF and DSS.

Warning signs that may occur at or after defervescence (the presence of one or more of these signs indicates the need for immediate medical evaluation):

- Abdominal pain or tenderness

- Persistent vomiting

- Clinical fluid accumulation (i.e., pleural effusion or ascites)

- Mucosal bleeding

- Lethargy or restlessness

- Liver enlargement ($\geq$2cm)

- Increases in hematocrit concurrent with rapid decrease in platelet count

Anticipatory management and monitoring indicators are essential in effectively administering therapies as the patient enters the Critical Phase. New-onset leucopenia (WBC <5,000 cells/mm3) with a lymphocytosis and an increase in atypical lymphocytes indicate that the fever will likely dissipate within the next 24 hours and that the patient is entering into the Critical Phase. Indicators that suggest the patient has already entered the Critical Phase include sudden change from high (>38.0°C) to normal or subnormal temperatures, thrombocytopenia ($\leq$100,000 cells/mm3) with a rising or elevated hematocrit ($\geq$20% increase from baseline), new hypoalbuminemia or hypocholesterolemia, new pleural effusion or ascites, and signs and symptoms of impending or frank shock.

Again, the key to successfully managing patients with DHF and lowering the probability of complications or death is early recognition and anticipatory treatment. Supportive care and timely but measured intravascular volume replacement during the Critical Period are the mainstays of treatment for DHF and DSS. (For more detailed guidance on management guidance, please see the recommended treatment courses for DHF in the links listed below link.)

Fortunately, the Critical Period lasts no more than 24 to 48 hours. Most of the complications that arise during this period--such as hemorrhage and metabolic abnormalities (e.g., hypocalcemia, hypoglycemia, hyperglycemia, lactic acidosis, and hyponatremia) are frequently related to prolonged shock. Hence, the principal objective during this period is to prevent prolonged shock and support vital systems until plasma leak subsides. Careful attention must be paid to the type of intravenous fluid (or blood product if transfusion is needed) administered, the rate, and the volume received over time. Frequent monitoring of intravascular volume, vital organ function, and the patient's response are essential for successful management during the Critical Phase. Monitoring for overt and occult hemorrhage (which may be another source of intravascular depletion) is also important. Transfusion of volume-replacing blood products should be considered if substantial hemorrhage is suspected during this phase. (For more detailed guidance on management, please see the recommended treatment courses for DHF in the links listed below.)

Convalescent (Reabsorption) Phase: The third phase begins when the Critical Phase ends and is characterized when plasma leak stops and reabsorption begins. During this phase, fluids that leaked from the intravascular space (i.e., plasma and administered intravenous fluids) during the Critical Phase are reabsorbed. Indicators suggesting that the patient is entering the Convalescent Phase include sense of improved well being reported by the patient, return of appetite, stabilizing vital signs (widen pulse pressure, strong palpable pulse), bradycardia, hematocrit levels returning to normal, increased urine output, and appearance of the characteristic Convalescence Rash of Dengue (i.e., a confluent sometimes pruritic, petechial rash with multiple small round islands of unaffected skin). At this point, care must be taken to recognize signs indicating that the intravascular volume has stabilized (i.e., that plasma leak has halted) and that reabsorption has begun. Modifying the rate and volume of intravenous fluids (and often times discontinuing intravenous fluids altogether) to avoid fluid overload as the extravasated fluids return to the intravascular compartment is important.

Complications that arise during Convalescent (Reabsorption) Phase are frequently related to the intravenous fluid management. Fluid overload may result from use of hypotonic intravenous fluids or over use or continued use of isotonic intravenous fluids during the Convalescence Phase... (For more detailed guidance on management please see the recommended treatment courses for DHF in the links listed below.)

Although an infected patient will likely have been very uncomfortable (from eye, joint, bone, muscle, or head pain) during the illness, barring complications such as fluid overload or mechanical ventilation nearly all patients with DHF recover rapidly with timely initiation of judicious fluid management and careful monitoring. This is due to the fact that the period of increased vascular permeability is time-limited (lasting 24 to 48 hours) and the functional change in the vascular endothelium appears to be entirely reversible with no known permanent structural defect. Even those with complications, if managed successfully, often recover fully without sequelae.

On-Line Dengue Course for Physicians

The US Centers for Disease Control has created **a free on-line course, in English and Spanish, for physicians** who need to familiarize themselves with Dengue diagnosis and treatment.

Goal

Provide information to enable physicians to recognize Dengue cases early in the clinical course, assess patients appropriately, and provide timely treatment.

Course Objectives

After completing this course, you will be able to

- Recognize and assess a patient with Dengue.

- Explain how the Dengue virus is transmitted, and list preventive measures.

- Describe the clinical course of Dengue, and explain WHO case definition.

- List diseases and conditions that are on the differential diagnosis of Dengue.

- Identify complications in each phase of the illness, and

- Explain how to recognize warning signs, plasma leakage, and early signs of shock.

- Demonstrate knowledge of how to apply correct treatment to Dengue patients.

Minimum System Requirements

- Microsoft® Internet Explorer® 7.0 browser (or higher) on standard Microsoft® technologies, i.e. Windows® NT®, Windows® 2000 or Mozilla Media™

- 233 MHz processor

- Windows® XP SP2

- JavaScript enabled

- Popup blocker disabled

- Intel® Pentium® III Processor

- 256 MB RAM

- Microsoft Windows® Media™ player for multimedia support

- RAM (for the browser alone): 64 MB for 32-bit Windows XP/Server 2003, 128 MB for 64-bit Windows XP/Server 2003

- Adobe® Flash® 7.6 plug-in software, compatible with the browser above

Link

Again, here's where to start the course.

More Clinical Guidelines for the Management of Dengue Infection

- WHO guidelines for the clinical management of Dengue infection 🗗

- WHO guidelines for treatment of Dengue fever/Dengue hemorrhagic fever in small hospitals PDF (234KB/33pages)
- Dengue case definition
- PDF CSTE Nationally Notifiable Condition List (10.7KB/2pages)
- Clinical management tools for health care providers
- Information for health care practitioners PDF(1.13MB/4pages)
- Requesting Dengue laboratory testing and case reporting
- Instructions for collecting, preparing and mailing specimens for Dengue testing at the CDC Dengue Laboratory PDF(134KB/7pages) and Spanish DOC (78KB/5pages)
- Hospitals, laboratories and health care centers in Puerto Rico that will draw serum samples (Spanish). DOC (104KB/1page)